NEW HOLLAND
PROFESSIONAL

MANICURE
AND PEDICURE

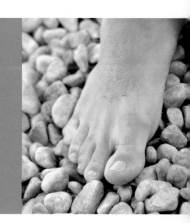

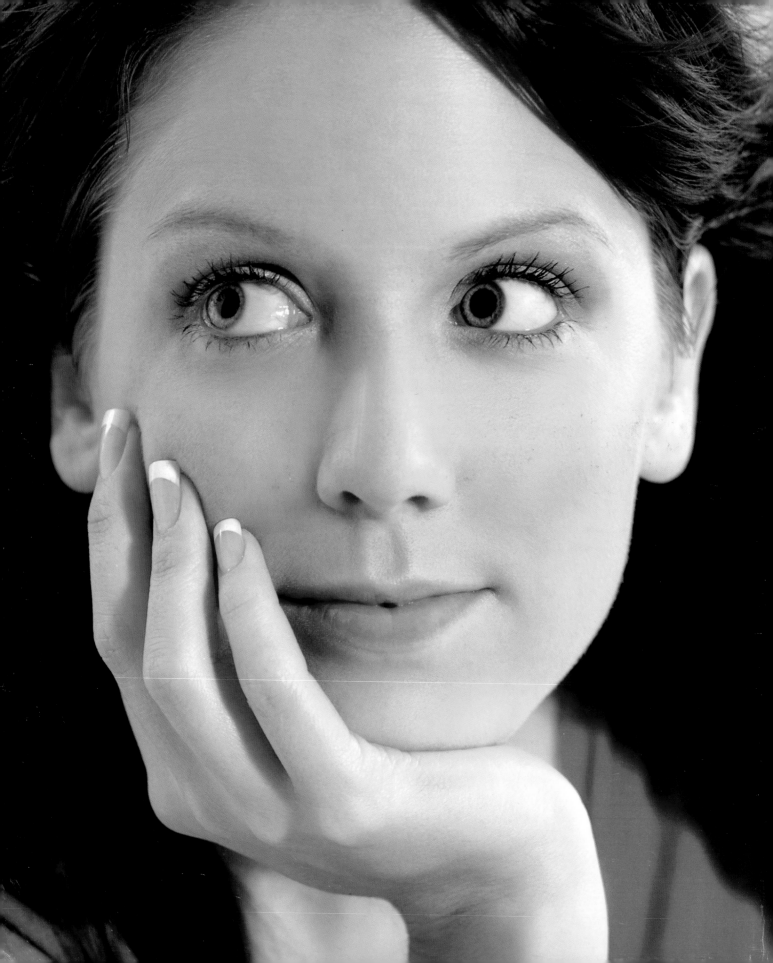

NEW HOLLAND

PROFESSIONAL

MANICURE AND PEDICURE

rosie watson

NEW HOLLAND

First published in 2008 by New Holland Publishers (UK) Ltd
London • Cape Town • Sydney • Auckland

Garfield House
86-88 Edgware Road
London W2 2EA
United Kingdom
www.newhollandpublishers.com

80 McKenzie Street
Cape Town 8001
South Africa

Unit 1
66 Gibbes Street
Chatswood
NSW 2067
Australia

218 Lake Road
Northcote
Auckland
New Zealand

ISBN 978 1 84537 977 3

Senior Editor **Corinne Masciocchi**
Designer **Isobel Gillan**
Photographer **Paul West**
Production **Marion Storz**
Editorial Direction **Rosemary Wilkinson**

10 9 8 7 6 5 4 3 2 1

Reproduction by Pica Digital PTE Ltd, Singapore
Printed and bound by Craft Print International Ltd, Singapore

contents

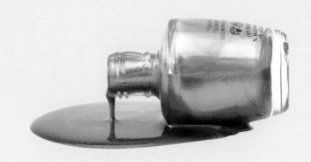

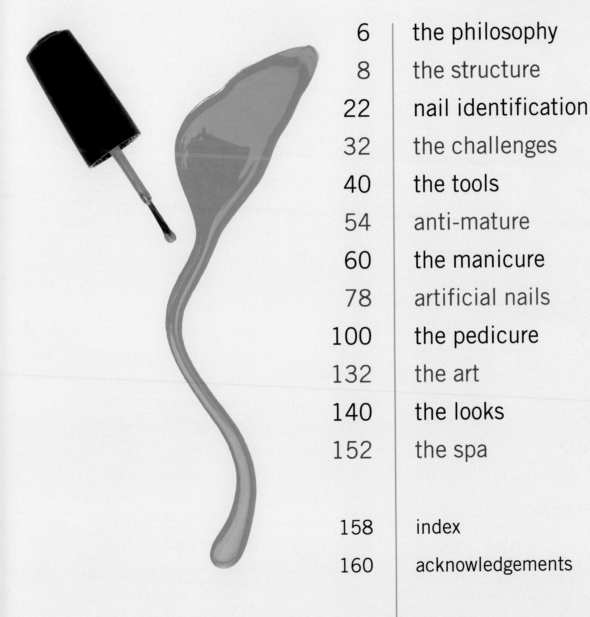

the philosophy

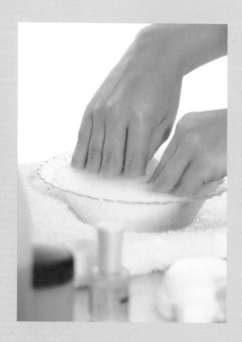

When I visited New York a few months ago, I realised what a growing industry the manicure and pedicure business was. New York was one of the first places to do nails on a large scale and the trend seems to have spread across the world like wildfire! I have noticed nail treatments growing in popularity in the salons in Britain and both my female and male clientele have expanded vastly in the last few years.

What I have seen in the nail bars in other nail progressive countries is a quick, clean and professional service for the price of a glass of wine! I realised that both women and men are now regularly having treatments, not just as an occasional treat but almost as a necessity, just like their regular dose of cappuccino!

Hands make the first touch when greeting someone new, in the form of a handshake. Hands show the world you have pledged your married life to someone with a wedding ring. Hands are kissed by others in some countries as a welcome and hands show some of the worst signs of stress in nail biters! So there is a clear emotional connection between us and our hands and nails. It is always good to look after hands and to appear well groomed at all times. The simplest manicure will revolutionise hands and nails and make us feel instantly better.

Feet, on the other hand, are rarely exposed but when they are they need to be shown to their full potential! Well groomed feet make all the difference and paying them a little attention provides fantastic results. Impressions are everything so why not let your body scream confidence all the way down to your toes?

It seems in modern day living you are now behind the times if your weekly schedule does not include a 45-minute appointment with a nail technician. It is rare for some to see the week through without either a manicure or a pedicure, even if it just a quick self-varnish.

If you haven't had a nail treatment before go to a nail bar and try it out! It is the right of all of us to treat ourselves once in a while and why not the hands and feet, which are often neglected and overlooked. We use them every day and having a warm wax or hot oil treatment, or wrapping them in warm mitts can really make a difference.

Currently fashions remain fairly similar to seasons past and the French style of varnish is still a favourite for making the nails look clean, fresh and well maintained. However, shorter dark nails are also coming into the limelight now and the vamp look is also very popular.

Colour should not be worn for fashion necessarily but to inspire the wearer and perhaps to match a particular outfit or accessory – this is when nail colour is at its most visually powerful! 'Sqoval' nails (nails with a tip in between square and oval) have been the height of fashion for many years but may not be to everyone's taste, so wear the nails you love regardless of fashions. You know what you like and it will be hard to feel comfortable wearing anything else.

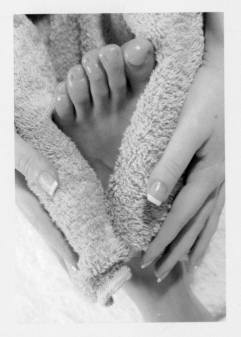

Rosie

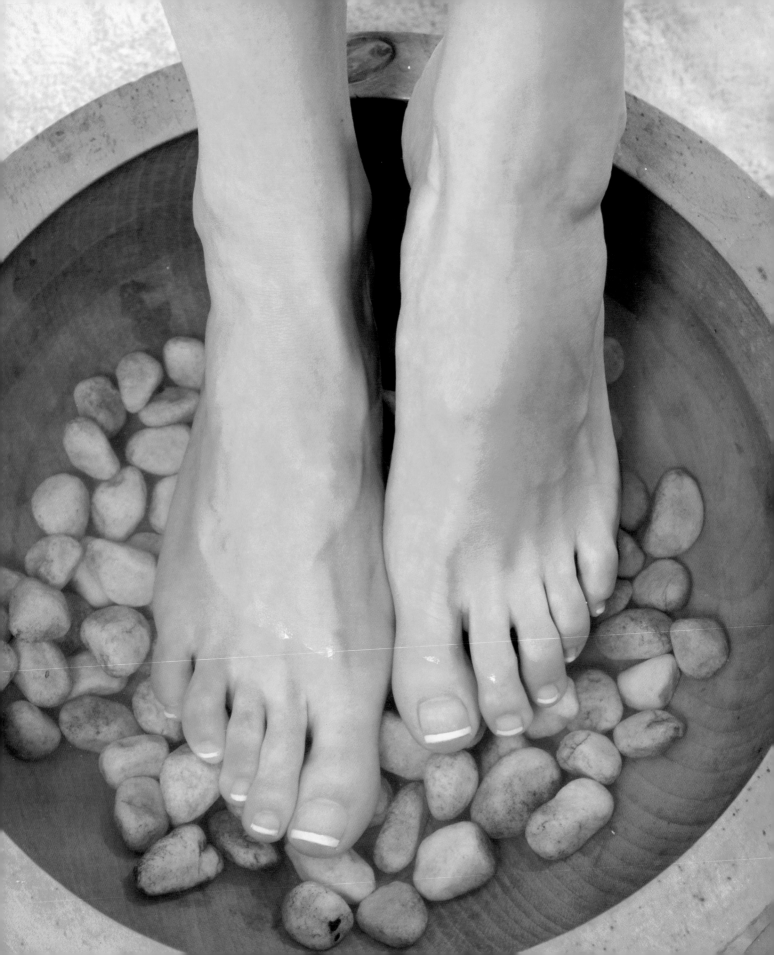

01 the structure

the structure

Having a manicure or pedicure these days is as popular as going for a coffee! In some cities it is unheard of to miss a nail appointment as the practice is now not merely a pampering treatment but a grooming necessity.

Our hands are used a great deal in communicating with others. We touch others with our hands and it is easy to make judgments on a person from the state of their hands and nails: bitten and they are stressed, pressurised and busy; too long and they have too much time to spare. Yellow nails scream out ill health, while dry hands suggest they do manual labour jobs and will be rough to touch. Why let people make assumptions before they have even spoken to you?

The hands and feet are known as body extremities and both these are prone to bad circulation and neglect. Feet can sometimes seem just that little too far away to reach and nail varnish takes longer to dry than we think we can afford! Physiologically feet need to be looked after well, especially as they support our whole body weight for many hours of the day, but hands, too, are in constant use and should be well looked after and regularly groomed. Investing a little time every week on our hands and feet makes all the difference.

The skin

Skin is made up of three main layers. The epidermis comprises the top set of five layers and is about as thick as a piece of paper; the dermis is the second main layer and is more complex in structure. The third is called the subcutaneous layer and is made up of fat cells.

The epidermis's main function is that of protection, as the top surface layers consist of dead skin cells and have no other direct function. Skin cells are constantly shed throughout the day and we lose hundreds of thousands every time we wash our hands, scratch or change clothes! The epidermis protects the underlying tissues from damage and also traps bacteria by secreting a sticky oil called sebum from glands deep in the hair follicle. Sebum is made up of cholesterol and acids and provides a natural moisturiser that gives suppleness to the skin. The acids are used to neutralise many types of bacteria and prevent internal infections. It is in the epidermis that we see physical ageing and the top visible layers of the skin can clearly mirror our inner imbalance or wellbeing.

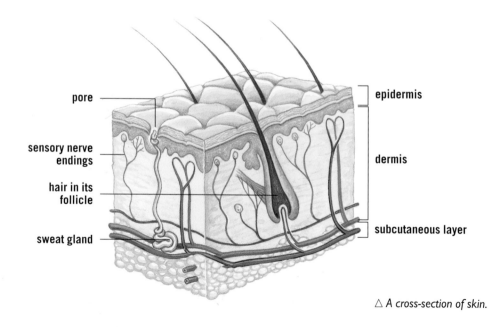

pore

sensory nerve endings

hair in its follicle

sweat gland

epidermis

dermis

subcutaneous layer

△ A cross-section of skin.

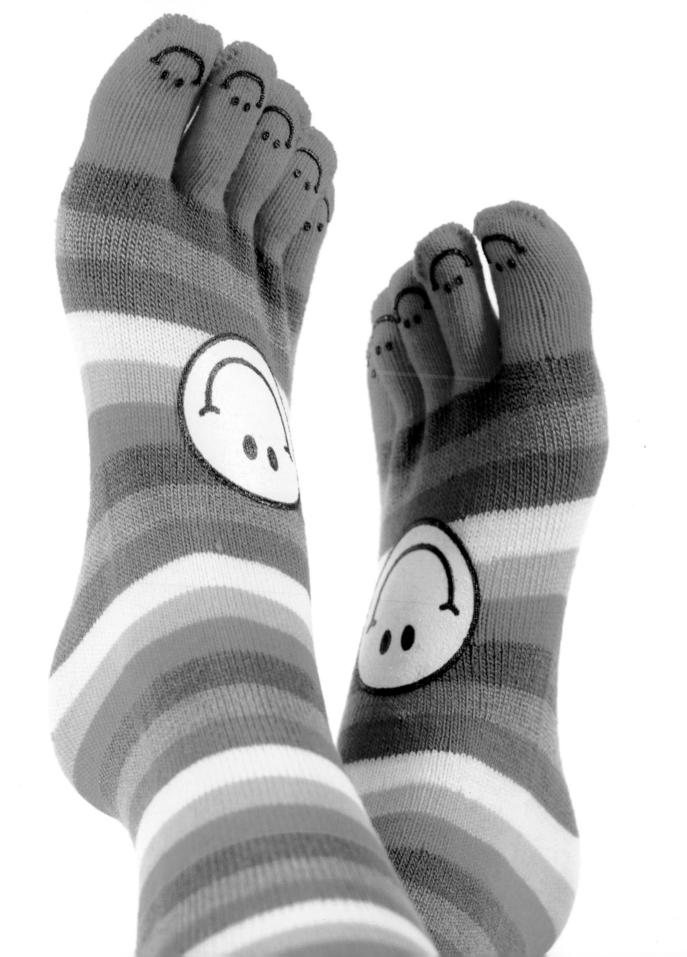

The epidermis's slightly acidic pH is about 5.5–6 and this protective, mildly acid mantel also helps to ward off harmful infections and bacteria. The epidermis on the palms of the hands and soles of the feet are the thickest in the body and are therefore one of the most protected areas.

Under the epidermis lies the dermis, a layer of skin made up of blood vessels and fibres such as collagen and elastin. It is subdivided into two layers and here is where skin cells are reproduced and grow. The tissue is fresh, new and plump. Collagen in this layer gives the skin a youthful appearance. Skin also needs to move and stretch and this is made possible by elastin found in the dermis. It is a stretchy fibre which allows great movement of the skin. With age, both collagen and elastin diminish in function and so visible ageing of the skin occurs.

Nutrients, oxygen and water, which are vital for skin maintenance, are distributed in the dermis by the blood stream, and nerve endings are also stored here so we can feel textures, heat, cold and pressure easily.

Under the dermis we find the last of the three main layers of the skin: the subcutaneous layer. It is basically made of fat cells which give the body warmth and protection against external damage. Some subcutaneous layers are deeper than others but this necessary layer also protects muscles and bones from damage as well as acting as the body's internal thermometer.

Together the epidermis and dermis weigh about 3 kg (7 lb), making skin the largest organ in the body. The skin combines together to form a very clever group of cells, as together they are responsible for protection, perspiration, sensation, heat regulation and excretion of unwanted bacterial invaders.

The back of the hands and feet have hair projections that trap air and keep us warm as well as being attached to senses which alert us to particles on the skin, as well as the heat or cold. This vellus hair can be very fine or very thick depending on nationality or hereditary genetics. The back of the hand is very susceptible to ageing, loose elastin and the breakdown of collagen, which, as time goes by, exaggerate the lines and wrinkles on our hands. The sun, too, damages skin texture, making it uneven and creating age or liver spots which once developed are very difficult to eradicate.

The nails

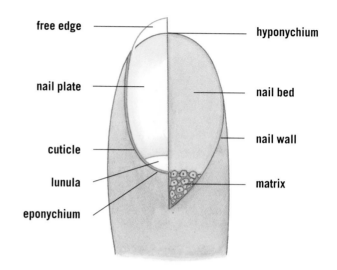

△ The basic anatomy of the nail.

All visible nail tissue is made of 'keratinised' particles (dead cells). Nails provide much protection from damage to the soft fingers and toe tips which we use constantly. Nails are translucent but colour can be seen as a faint pink from the blood supply beneath the nails, or they can also turn blue with cold or ill health.

It takes about six months to grow a nail from its root (the matrix) to the free edge at the end of the fingertip and this regular growth means we have to cut, file and buff our nails regularly. The longest nails in history are about 76 cm (30 in) long but most of us like to maintain a comfortable workable length of a few millimetres!

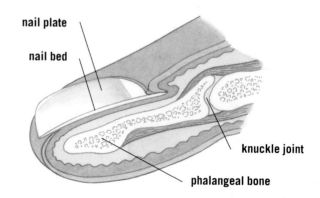

△ A cross-section of a finger.

- **Massaging the matrix of the nail increases blood supply and helps to speed up the production of new nail cells to increase growth speed.**

- **Warm hand treatments should be concentrated around the matrix as increased heat will improve circulation to the nails and make them look pinker and healthier.**

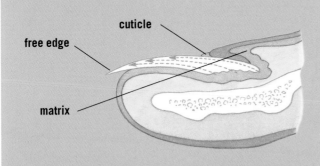

cuticle

free edge

matrix

△ *Nails are always slightly curved to give them exceptional strength and durability.*

The technical name for a nail is an 'onyx' and it is usually flat and slightly pink in colour with an opaque edge at the fingertip. As it is made of keratinised cells we can manipulate the texture and shape of the nails without any pain or discomfort. Hot water and chemicals will soften the nail's structure and allow flexibility whereas cold water will encourage the nail to retain the same structure and limited flexibility.

The matrix of the nail is more commonly known as the root and this is the only area where the nail is alive and reproduces new nail cells. A healthy blood supply to the matrix brings life-giving oxygen and nutrition to new nail cells. Subsequently, a healthy matrix will lead to a healthy nail. However, if the matrix is damaged, the nail may grow abnormally or not at all.

The half moon (lunula) of the nail is visible at the top of the matrix and the base of the nail plate. This narrow crescent is slightly white in colour because the new nail cells are compacting down to become stronger and this process cuts out the visibility of the underlying blood supply which gives nails their pink appearance. The lunula was said to show how long you would live and how healthy you are but

the size of your lunula is not relevant to age nor health! Some people have no visible lunula yet stay alive! In the early days of the French manicure, nail technicians used to paint the lunula as well as the free edge of the nails white but this fashion died as the complexity of this work was too great for everyday wear.

The nail bed is the area of flesh that lies under the nail plate and contains the blood vessels that give nails their healthy pink colour. The nail bed contains small ridges to provide extra adherence to the nail plate and is the area we see if we lose the nail plate in an accident.

The nail plate makes up the whole surface of the nail we see and feel. It is hard and made of compacted dead cells. It is usually slightly shiny and is stuck fast to the nail bed on which it lies. The nail plate can grow very long past the finger's edge and when the plate is no longer stuck to the nail bed the plate becomes the 'free edge'. This free edge is the area we class as the nail's length and is usually white or opaque in colour as there is no pink from underlying tissues to be seen through it.

The cuticle of the nail is the rim of skin lying from the nail matrix around the base and sides of the nail. Its purpose is to protect the matrix from invading bacteria and water which

- **When cleaning beneath the nail's free edge do so gently or you could damage the delicate skin that joins the nail plate to the nail bed, thus reducing the surface area of the nail bed! In the long term this can lead to the lifting of the plate as well as possible infections or discomfort.**

- **Gently buffing the nails with a fine-grain buffer will help to smooth unsightly ridges but be sure not to over-buff as the nails will just become thinner and weaker.**

- **A soft leather shimmy can really make the nails shine like they have varnish on so if your profession does not allow nail varnish try this instead for the same look!**

trade secrets

- Treating cuticles regularly with a massage oil or hand cream will help keep them pliable, and gently pushing them back weekly will keep them out of the way without having to cut them off completely.

- Long or unruly cuticles need to be trimmed with cuticle nippers to prevent the skin tearing which can be very painful and take a while to heal.

- Always warm the cuticles in warm water before treating them as they will expand and soften slightly in water.

- Keeping cuticles soft not only looks good but also prevents hang nails, which appear as loose, torn cuticles (pterygium) on the sides of the nails. If left these can become painful and unsightly.

could harm the growth of the nail. The cuticle is made of skin cells and if unkempt can grow far up the nail plate, producing unnecessary and unsightly protection. Contemporary fashions insist on pushing back the cuticle to make the lunula more visible and to increase the surface area of the nail plate for nail varnish application but it is essential not to over treat the cuticles as their function of protection is vital to maintain a healthy looking nail plate. Cutting the cuticle off completely can leave the nail's surface and matrix open to infections and can increase the bulk of the cuticle as it grows back.

Anatomy

One of the best parts of a hand or foot treatment is the massage. When applied correctly this series of stroking and kneading movements can evoke deep relaxation and tension release and it is all down to the bones, muscles and nerves in the hands and feet!

Bone tissue is strong and when used all the time, as with the hands and feet, the joints that link the bones together can become stiff and painful. Massaging around the bones can loosen the joints and muscles which lie in between the bones.

THE HANDS

The bones in the hands are grouped into three categories: the carpals, which are the bones found in the wrist; the metacarpals, those in the palm of the hand; and the phalanges, which are the finger bones. The muscles are interlinked with bones to give power and strength to our grasp and pull movements. Along with the muscles in the hands which enable a plethora of movements, the arms and shoulders are also involved with most hand movements and therefore should be massaged alongside the hands and wrists.

The complex nerve network in the hands comprises sensory nerves that lie under the skin allowing us to feel pain, heat and pressure. Motor nerves carry messages from the brain and spine to the hands to activate the muscles to move. When treated with massage both motor and sensory nerve endings are stimulated and soothed to enforce relaxation.

BONES

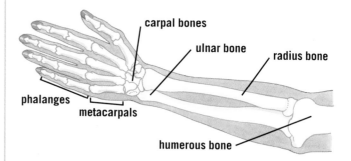

carpal bones
ulnar bone
radius bone
phalanges
metacarpals
humerous bone

MUSCLES

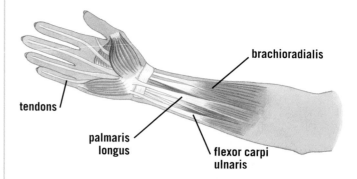

brachioradialis
tendons
palmaris longus
flexor carpi ulnaris

△ *When massaging, remember to massage around the bones, too.*

THE FEET

The bones in the feet are also grouped into three categories: the tarsal bones are the ankle bones; the metatarsals are the bones making up the sole of the foot; and the phalanges are the bones in the toes. The nineteen muscles that make up the foot help us to achieve balance, run, walk and stand in various positions. The muscle and nerve structures are similar to those of the hands and will therefore have a similar effect when treated with massage. Often though, feet can be susceptible to foot problems as more often than not we may feel they are too far away to bother with!

Nail therapy

Nail treatments are not only designed to make the nails look groomed, they contain ingredients designed for pure pampering, and the deeper tissues of the skin, muscles and bones are stimulated and affected. Joints can be mobilised and skin complaints treated as well as circulation increased to bring warmth to the extremities and increase the feeling of wellbeing. Massage can be very invigorating but other forms of manipulation can be used to treat zones in the body that have specific energy functions. Treatments like reflexology, reiki, and trigger point massage are a few which work really well on the hands and feet and have the added advantage of being preformed pretty much anywhere!

REFLEXOLOGY

Reflexology is an age-old treatment on the hands and feet to treat other areas of the body through various pressure points found on the palms and soles. The diagram below shows a 'body map' of the palms and soles.

Before commencing a reflexology session, warm the hands or soles first to increase blood circulation and enforce warmth on to the colder areas. After this warming massage, apply pressure to the area you wish to treat, slowly at first, then once pressure has been applied, complete a series of pumping movements to increase the effectiveness of the treatment. Apply small circular movements as you gently release the pressure from the pressure point. For a quick fix at work, the hands are a more practical option but when relaxing at home the more powerful effects will be felt from a foot treatment.

If you are not sure which organs are responsible for what, consult the anatomy guide below for the low-down on organ function.

▽ *Pressure points enduce holistic therapy and pure relaxation.*

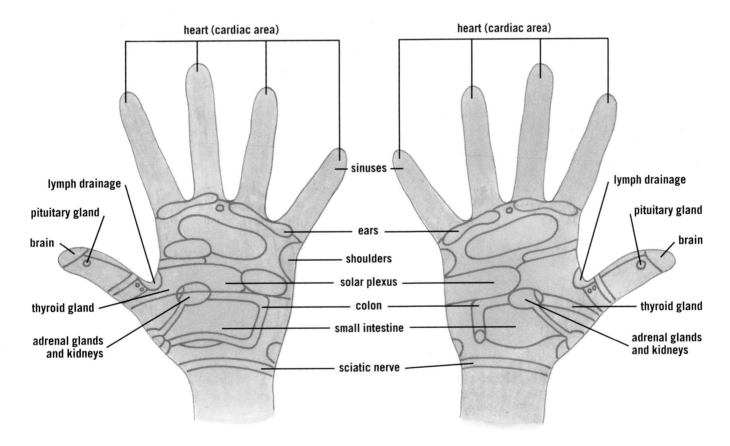

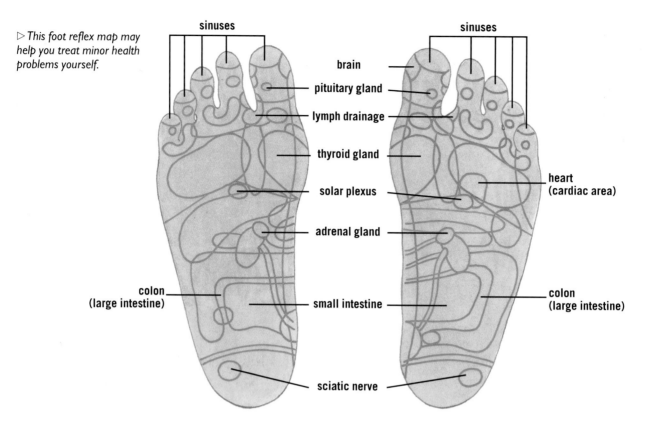

▷ This foot reflex map may help you treat minor health problems yourself.

Labels on image: sinuses, sinuses, brain, pituitary gland, lymph drainage, thyroid gland, solar plexus, adrenal gland, heart (cardiac area), colon (large intestine), small intestine, colon (large intestine), sciatic nerve

All reflexology treatments treat the body holistically and indirectly help to relieve pressure in the body and release the symptoms of psychosomatic illness (physical illness caused or influenced by emotional factors and stress). Examples of these illnesses are headaches, backache, excessive perspiration, eye strain and anxiety. Ongoing illness or pain should always be treated by a doctor before self treatment is applied with foot or hand massage and pressure points. However, 'self reflexology' can be very relaxing: link the pressure points shown above with these common ailments:

Sinuses Found under the forehead bone, sinuses go from the top of the nose to the forehead and at the sides of the head, and when blocked feel like pressure around the eyes and nose. Sinuses are like fingerprints and are different for everyone. They can become painful with infection, colds and viruses so apply pressure to fingertips or toe tips to help release that bunged up feeling or discomfort in this area.

Lymph drainage Lymph is a substance that travels around the body, clearing it of toxins and waste. Light pressure applied at the base of the big toe space or in the thumb space will stimulate detoxification of the body and help reduce swelling in the body tissues if you suffer from puffy feet.

The brain Some headaches are thought to be caused by blood flowing incorrectly around the brain causing pain in different areas of the head. Reflexology here may well soothe a headache. Apply a slight pressure to the tip and side of the thumb or big toe to relieve symptoms.

Pituitary gland This endocrine gland is responsible for secreting important hormones which keep the body working and balanced. If hormone levels are unbalanced you may feel lethargic, sick, dehydrated and generally unwell. A light pressure applied to the point just below the thumbprint or at the base of the big toe will help balance problematic hormones.

Adrenal glands Treat these when stressed as the hormones adrenalin and cortisol produced by these glands are responsible for the 'fight or flight' mechanism which kicks in in times of stress. Pressure applied in the centre of the foot or hand can help to relax and calm from the inside out.

Thyroid gland This butterfly shaped gland in the neck region is responsible for regulating the body's metabolic rate, so if you feel unusually tired or hyperactive apply pressure on the inner upper foot area or at the base of the thumb.

Solar plexus This is known as the centremost part of the body and feelings of negativity and stress can be released when applying pressure in the centre of the palms and soles.

Small intestine This is where most of the food in our body is absorbed and digested to use for energy. Irritable Bowel Syndrome (IBS) and other digestive complaints such as diarrhoea or constipation may be soothed with a light thumb pressure on the lower inside of the soles and centre of the palms.

Colon This is the waste carrier and the tube that carries faeces to the anus. Bowl problems and constipation are treated with pressure points to the 'C' shaped area found in the lower part of the soles and palms.

Cardiac area This area is responsible for the heart and blood circulation so any problems with nervous anxiety or bad circulation can be treated by applying pressure to the upper central sole and upper left palm.

Sciatic nerve This is the largest nerve in the body and it runs from the very bottom of the back down the outside of the thigh and leg. It can be painful if trapped and cause untold problems. Soothing pressure points at the very bottom of the heal and wrist can help relieve some of the pain.

Shoulders We all have tense, tight shoulders but cannot massage them directly ourselves but the next best thing is using the pressure points on your hands to treat them indirectly. Massage all over the palms and pressure points around the pads of the palms for tension release.

Reflexology on the feet is regularly used to treat other parts of the body and training a partner or family member to massage your feet is well worth the effort! The pressure points on the feet are similar to those on the hands but because the sole is a larger area it can be easier to treat.

The hands and feet have an exceptionally rich supply of blood and nerve endings. This gives them the ability to be very sensitive and functional as well as warm and strong. When treating the hands and feet it is always better to work with massage movements running towards the top of the arms and the top of the legs as these areas are closer to the heart. By encouraging this flow of blood and lymphatic waste

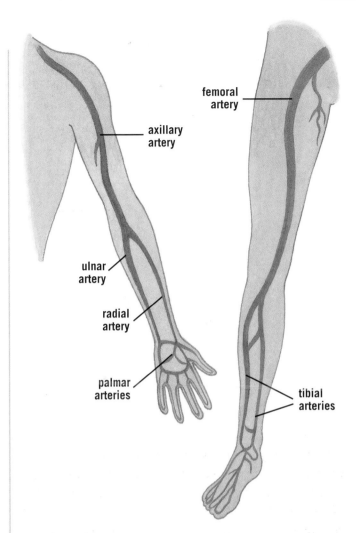

△ *Massaging stimulates the blood supply which turns the skin pink. This is known as 'erythema'.*

upwards you are stimulating those systems to work more efficiently and quickly.

Though the muscles in the hands and feet can be very strong they are very delicately structured. Muscles help retain heat from the blood and keep the extremities warm

THE PROFESSIONAL TOUCH

It is always better to receive treatment from a qualified reflexologist and the recommendations set out here are for a temporary self-treatment fix only. Should you feel unwell or have a condition that needs medical attention, seek the advice of a medically trained person before proceeding with self treatment.

even when they are not being used. As a masseuse your hand muscles can become exceptionally strong and so exercising them is useful. Hand and foot exercises are great to do as part of a nail treatment at home to relax and warm the muscles as well as mobilising joints and nerves to help prevent repetitive strain injuries.

Nature

Improving the appearance of nails without the use of products can be effectively done by following a good exercise regime to constantly increase the blood supply to the growth zones of the nails. A good diet will be high in nail nourishment like vitamins A, B, C, D and E as well as minerals like zinc and magnesium which boost nail strength. Protecting the nails from chemicals and cleaning fluids helps keep their appearance glowing and a good trim now and again will maintain their shape and prevent splitting and peeling.

Nurture

Other than the above most of us require a little more from our nails than just functionality. There is nothing wrong with adding a little pampering pizzazz into your life with a lovely nail treatment and a vibrant colour to finish! So out with the norm and on with the fabulous!

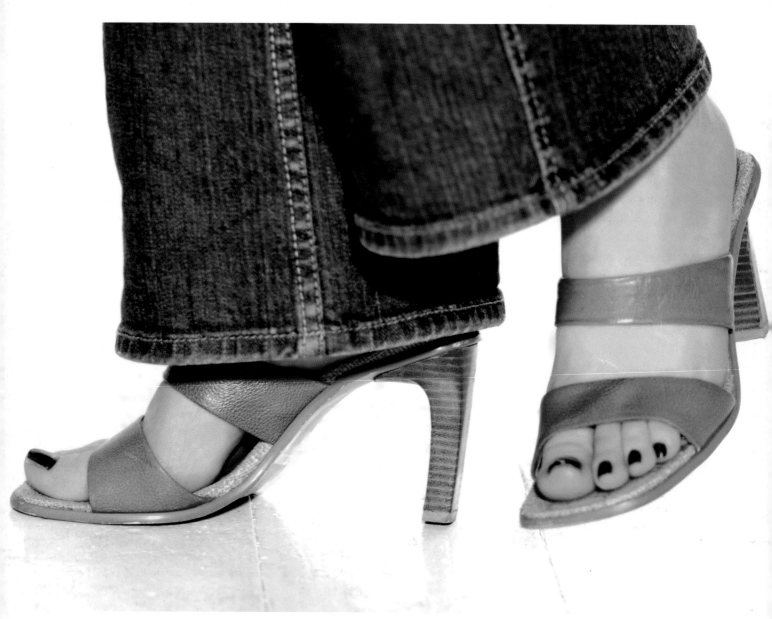

THE FOOT GYM

Feet can easily become tired, puffy and painful. These exercises help relax muscles and mobilise joints in the feet, aiding relaxation especially after wearing high heels all day!

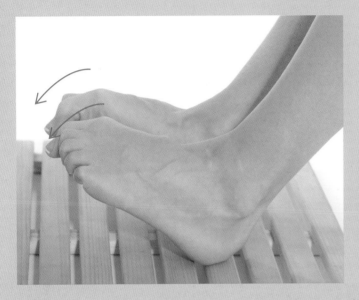

① Scrunching up and flexing the toes is the best way to exercise the phalanges, enabling freer movement of the toes.

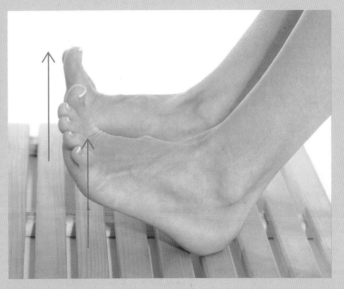

② You will do this instinctively after wearing high heeled shoes but a regular phalange stretch works wonders for relaxation of toe muscles.

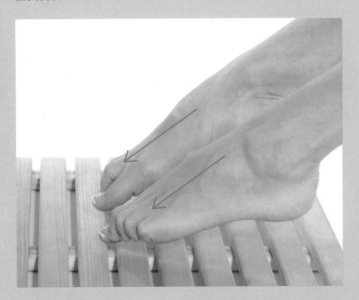

③ Pointing the toes is a great foot relaxer, too. Just be a little careful about quick movements as this can cause cramp in the toes which is uncomfortable!

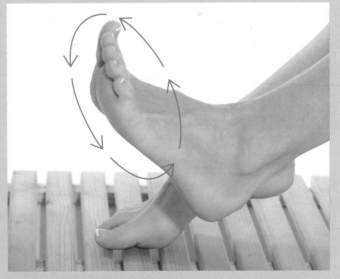

④ Foot circles can really manipulate the tarsal joints in the ankle and help with lower leg swelling. Rotate the foot to the extremities of its capabilities but ensure no pain is felt.

THE HAND GYM

With age, illness or even just cold weather, joints can get stiff and painful. Try these simple hand exercises before carrying out a manicure to awaken tired joints and loosen tight muscles.

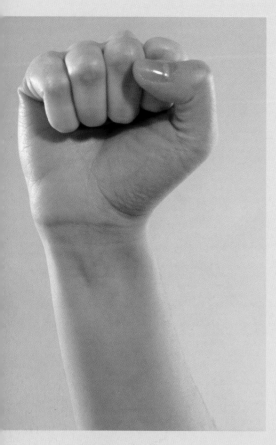

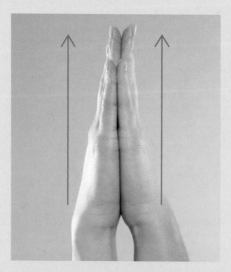

② Place hands in the prayer position.

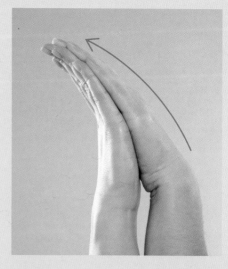

③ Apply pressure to each set of fingers in turn...

① Make a fist with your hands and squeeze as hard as you can to increase strength in your wrists and fingers. Repeat nine more times.

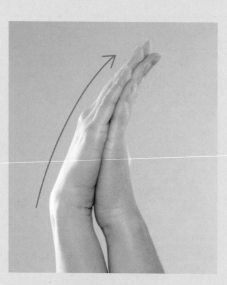

④ ... to stretch the base of the fingers without putting pressure on the knuckles.

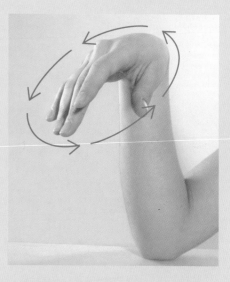

⑤ Wrist rotating is good for mobilising the carpal joints but be sure to do this slowly and if pain occurs cease the action immediately.

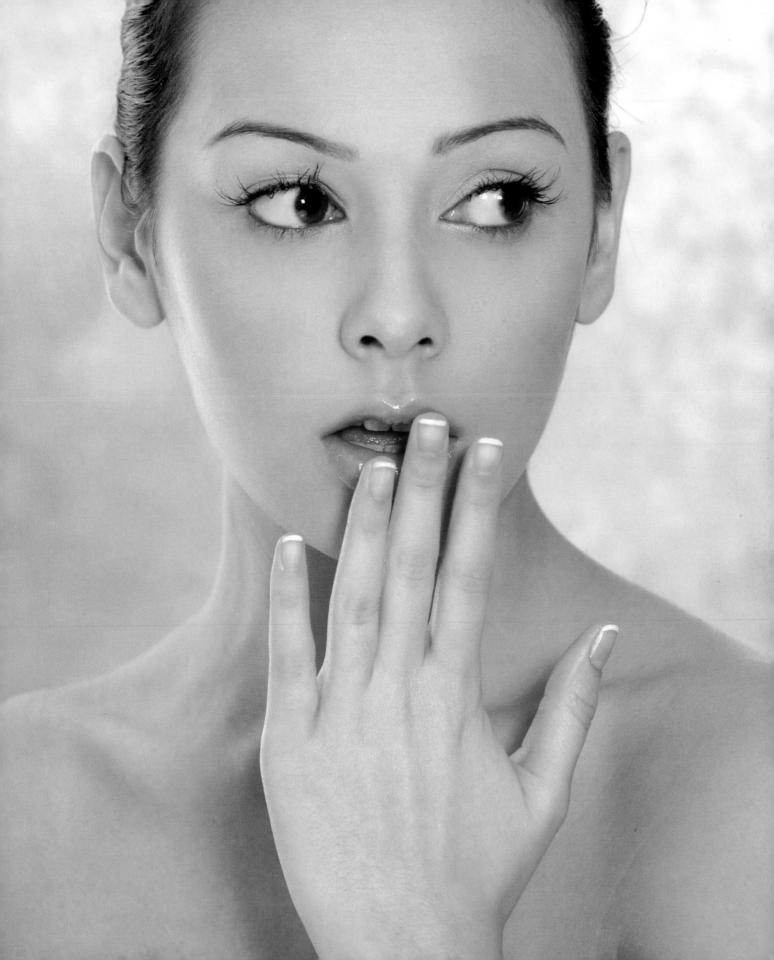

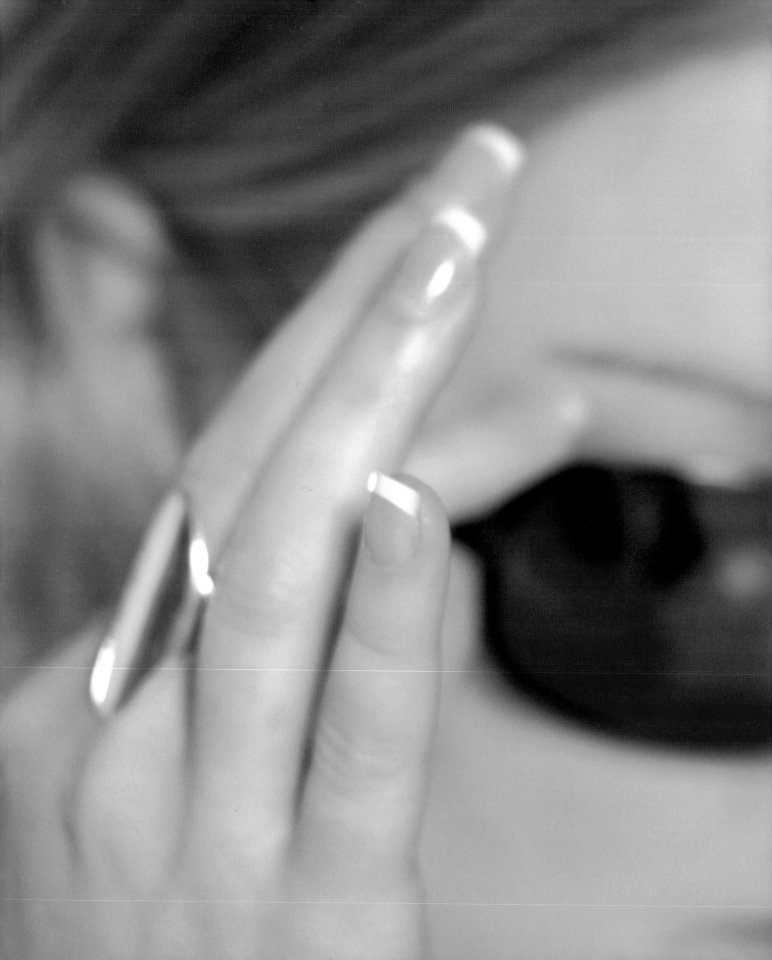

02 nail identification

nail identification

Nails carry out many basic functions. They predominantly act as tools, providing a strong surface to utilise for opening and levering packages as well as picking, scratching and all manner of tasks. Nails can be used as weapons, too, but breaking one perfect talon will anger you far more than the initial problem and take longer to repair!

Nails are made of hard compacted dead cells which form a firm but flexible surface. In this era of innutritious diets, overwork and stress our nails feel the pressure too and can appear to be unwell. This manifests itself as flaking, peeling or dryness, to name a few symptoms. Treatments are readily available now to help regenerate nails and deal with these problems, which can be unsightly and uncomfortable. We do not help our nails by using harsh chemicals without wearing protective gloves or constantly wearing nail extensions, so make sure you protect your nails and give them regular breaks from extensions.

There are nail types just like there are skin types and it is important to understand why you have a specific nail type and how to best treat the nails. Only then can you treat the nails properly and get the best look you can naturally.

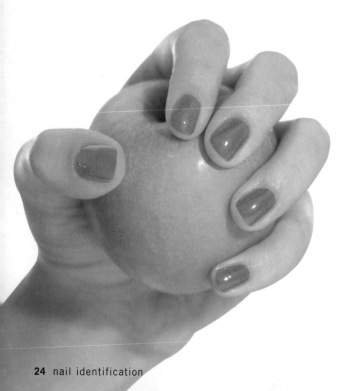

Natural nails look their best when they are clean and well groomed. Often nails that are too long are in danger of breaking or splitting and generally need more maintenance. Look for a quick and easy solution to rebalance the nails either by adding more moisture to the nails in the form of an oil applied to soften them or by using nail hardening treatments to toughen them, then work to create the length and image you want.

Dry nails

Dry nails appear dull and may have superficial ridges, with dry cuticles and the skin on the fingertips dehydrated. The nails may peel easily and can readily flake on the free edge. Some dry nails appear thicker than usual due to the excessive build up of keratinised cells on the nail plate. Using strong cleaning detergents and bleach without wearing protective gloves dries the nails. Cold weather conditions can also lead to this exposed area suffering from a severe lack of moisture. Finally, short- or long-term illness, and a lack of fatty acids in the diet can make nails appear drier.

Dry nails tend to be made worse by an overuse of nail varnish remover as its high alcohol content strips the natural oil moisture from the nails. Over buffing and frequent use of artificial nails can make dry nails very brittle and they can shatter easily.

Remember that dryness is a lack of oil, not water, in the skin and nails so increase the use of oil-based hand and cuticle creams to treat this condition. Very dry hands and nails can crack and cause severe pain so don't forget to moisturise on a regular basis.

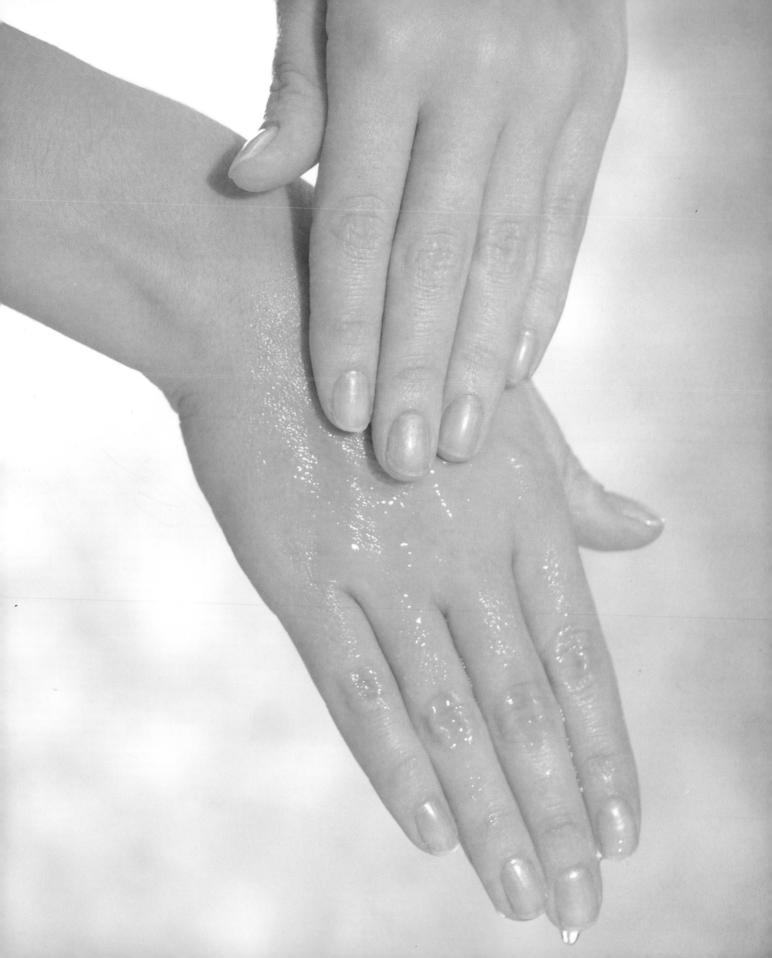

INTERNAL NAIL THERAPY

Dry nails respond well to a good injection of oil in the form of fatty acids which are found in evening primrose oil and olive oil. Vegetable oils in general help to support the wall of cells so when the nail cells are growing they will lose less moisture.

EXTERNAL NAIL THERAPY

Remember that dry nails crave moisture so treat them regularly with a nail oil or cream rubbed into the skin and cuticles surrounding the nail. Done on a daily basis this will help to soften the skin and decrease the chances of flaking and peeling of the nails and cuticles. Warm oil and wax treatments are really beneficial so a monthly spa treatment will really boost the nails and protect them against harsh environmental factors which could contribute to extra dryness.

Brittle nails

Brittle nails are distinguished by texture rather than appearance. They are very hard and tend to be slightly thicker than balanced nails. Because they are inflexible they shatter and break very easily and although they can reach long lengths they also tend to grow with a curve or at an odd angle after a certain length.

Brittle nails tend to look dry and have a dull surface, often caused by regular exposure to harsh chemicals either through cleaning or work-based activity and over-zealous use of nail varnish remover.

Brittle nails can often be caused by the use of too much nail strengthener. Soft nails can be made very hard with nail strengthening products but brittle is one stage further than necessary! Stop using these hardening products when your nails feel strong but still slightly flexible.

Because brittle nails tend to be dry and dehydrated they need to be treated with both oil- and water-based products as well as protectors to ensure moisture is not lost. Any loss of moisture will only dry the nails and make them harder which brittle nails definitely do not need!

If brittle nails do shatter, they tend to break very low on the nail plate, which will need a nail repair to grow out safely.

INTERNAL NAIL THERAPY

Vitamins work wonders for brittle nails especially vitamins C, D and E, all of which help to prevent thickening and discolouration of nails as well as increasing the absorption of other nutrients to help make the nails more flexible whilst maintaining their much needed strength. Increasing your water intake will increase hydration and help nails look pinker.

EXTERNAL NAIL THERAPY

A combination of extra oils, moisture and water-based products is necessary to re-flex brittle nails so treat them with warm nail treatments and massage regularly with hand cream or cuticle oil to prevent those shattering moments! Use conditioning nail varnish remover as it contains less alcohol and keep the nails short to prevent cracking.

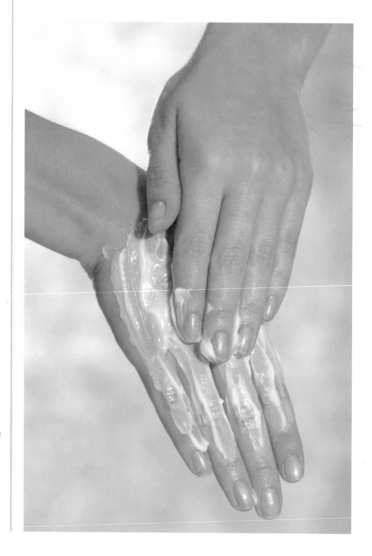

Dehydrated nails

Dehydrated nails are very different to dry nails. Dehydration is caused by a lack of water, not oil, in the nails and so they appear dull and can peel easily. These nails are often thinner and weaker than dry nails but still have the matt, flaky appearance of dry nails.

Often, dehydrated nails can deteriorate with age and mature nails often suffer from some dehydration. As we get older, a less rich supply of hormones, nutrients and proteins circulate in the blood. As fewer of these life-giving properties reach their source, the nail matrix, the nails will show themselves as lacking in moisture, water and nutrients.

Bad circulation in the hands and feet can also lead to dehydration in the nails and whether hereditary or developed, bad circulation can also give dehydrated nails a yellowy or blue appearance.

As we age, nails tend to grow more slowly due to the lack of circulating nutrients. To rejuvenate nail cells and boost their reproduction it is essential to prevent dehydration and increase blood circulation whenever possible to the fingers and toes and ultimately the nails themselves with daily massage.

INTERNAL NAIL THERAPY

All the vitamin Bs are best here and B2, B7 and B12 are the ones to take as they give strength to the nail cells being formed and nourish the matrix of the nail, increasing the chances of nutrient absorption and therefore healthier nails. Calcium is a mineral we ingest less with age but it is essential for maintaining healthy nails and skin as well as bones. Calcium is found primarily in dairy products and it can be taken in pill form.

EXTERNAL NAIL THERAPY

Dehydrated nails need extra care compared to other nail conditions as there are a number of treatments needed. Firstly a good water-based hand lotion applied regularly will be greatly appreciated by these nails and a surface cream mask and exfoliator will brighten the skin on the hands and help slough off stray nail cells which can make the nails look flaky. Regular water consumption will really boost the hydration of the blood and subsequently the nails, and a regular hand and nail massage will increase circulation to the fingers and nails, improving their chances of balance.

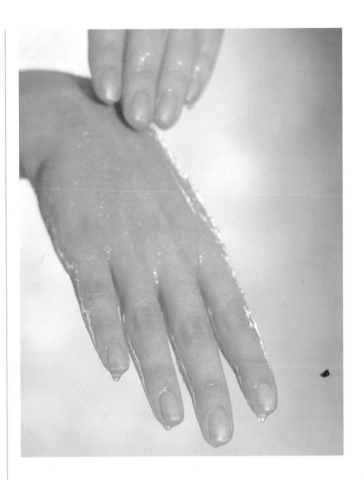

SOS damaged nails

Damage to nails can come from many sources such as illness, medication, over treatment, badly applied nail extensions, ill treatment of nails or harsh working environments. Unhealthy nails all have common traits: they appear weak, thin, over flexible and peel easily, and are slow to grow. They can often also seem dry and dehydrated, making this the hardest condition to recover from, but providing the best results when you do!

Thin nails are difficult to grow because they inevitably break or peel under daily pressure; they need protecting by treatment constantly until they can survive on their own. Good nutrition will help lay down strong cell foundations for growing nails to become strong and flexible.

The sun can damage nails, too, and lifestyle choices such as smoking and drinking alcohol will discolour the nails. This discolouration will have to grow out rather than being reduced by products or treatment. Dry skin and nails can exacerbate damaged nails and the more moisture they receive the better they will eventually look.

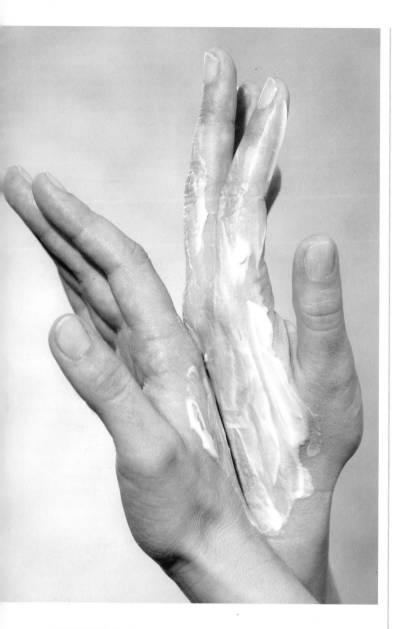

If a nail breaks repair it quickly and this stop gap measure will hopefully prevent a low and painful tear developing in the nail.

Tantalising tips

Every so often we come across those with stunning natural nails. Few and far between, these ten-fingered fancies put most of us to shame. But what is it that makes their nails so amazing to look at?

Firstly they have a natural pink undertone to the nail bed, suggesting good nutrient delivery from the blood and great circulation. Secondly they have a white free edge which appears to be a brilliant French manicure naturally! And thirdly they tend to have long, slender fingers and youthful hands to show off their slender youthful nails!

But the secret to nails that look great naturally are long nail plates – the longer the nail plate the more nail you have to look at. It is irrelevant how long the actual nails are as the plate is the area attached to the nail bed and therefore the area that looks healthy. The more you see of it the better the nails look.

Whether we possess long nail plates or not, making the most of our natural nails is essential, and this is to bring them as close to balance as normal. 'Normal' nails are strong, pink and flexible with a smooth surface and an unbreakable free edge.

Rising to perfection

Aside from treating nails with products and treatments we use our nails in everyday situations which can damage them. Simple steps and changes can prevent this from happening and you can still do the washing up!

TALON TIPS

★ Try not to use your nails as tools for opening tins or peeling off labels; your nails will inevitably peel, so use other items or get someone else to do it for you!

★ Wear protective gloves when gardening, cleaning, washing up and handling detergents, bleach and other strong chemicals. These strong substances ravage the natural oils in the nails and sap them of hydration, too. Some say it is difficult to feel or pick up things when wearing gloves but super thin latex gloves protect the nails and allow maximum movement too, so try them out!

INTERNAL NAIL THERAPY

Vitamin A and calcium are two of the best vitamins and minerals to combat damage to the nails as they increase growth and firm up nails naturally. A balanced diet can also contribute to balanced nail types and even though it may take a month to see the results they will be clear.

EXTERNAL NAIL THERAPY

Weak nails need care and moisture so keep them well protected by using regular treatments to improve flexibility and strength. Hand and nail treatments and masks are great for propelling ingredients into the surrounding skin tissue and improving the overall look of the hands and feet.

★ Try to keep nails short as they often look much better as well as being easier to maintain with a dramatic decrease in the chances of splitting and peeling.

★ Carry a nail file board with you everywhere as when a chip or break occurs a few wisps of the board will prevent picking and biting off too much nail! Nail clippers and nippers leave a harsh finish to the nails so it is vital to file these prospective sharp weapons into a smooth shape.

★ Vitamins are essential for good nail growth but increasing your levels of minerals and proteins will show vast improvements, too.

★ A mini manicure once a week will show just the right amount of care, and regular hand cream usage really boosts the appearance of the skin on the hands and feet as well as vitally boosting circulation to the growth zones of the nails.

★ Always use an acetone-free nail varnish remover to prevent too much drying on the surface of the nail. Try not to use remover more than once a week as over time the nails will become dry and brittle.

★ If you doubt the strength of your nails and worry about peeling even if they are short apply varnish to combat damage and protect the delicate surface of the nails. Varnish can be used regularly to protect the nails. Choosing a light or clear colour will make the nails look healthier as well as avoiding unwanted attention.

Problematic nails

Nails suffer from classic problems which we all suffer from at one time or another. These are simply unavoidable irritations caused by the work we do, the environment and even free radical damage (natural airborne unstable oxygen particles causing damage to the skin, hair and nails).

HERE'S HOW TO COPE!

Splitting nails Usually caused by dryness and external trauma, such as banging. Nails should not regularly split but if they do it is mainly due to a dysfunction at the matrix where the nail grows. As the nail grows up the plate there will likely be a weak spot which splits the nail when it reaches the free edge. To prevent this happening, nourish the cuticle to increase nutrient release from the blood which will make the nail grow stronger and more flexible. Using a strengthening base or a fibre-rich product will also help to hold and bind the surface of the nail together, preventing splitting. Worse case scenario, treat the nail with an invisible wrap to keep the length but stop the split! Nail glue can work wonders but apply only a small amount and hold in place with a pair of tweezers to prevent fingers sticking together! Finally keep the nails short as they will still look groomed and maintained but there will be a 50 per cent less chance of splitting occurring.

▽ *Nail treatments vary from strengtheners to fillers and softeners. Diagnose your nail type correctly and these miracle treatments will naturally complement your nails.*

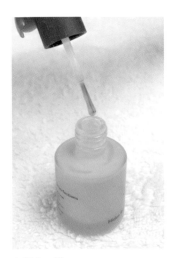

△ *Splitting nail treament.*

△ *Ridge filler treament.*

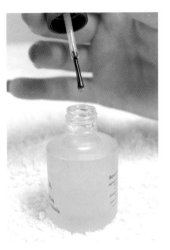

△ *Thin nail treament.*

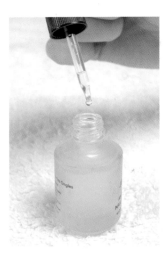

△ *Fungal infection treatment.*

Thin nails Normally a problem recognised by those of us with damaged or dehydrated nails, thin nails need protection and strength, so a good strengthening base coat will help to build up firmness whilst applying a clear or coloured varnish will protect the nails from external damage while they grow. Be sure to avoid constant usage of strengthening products as they can make the nails brittle but over a short period of time they can work well. Again, keep the nails short while you treat them and when they begin to grow thicker you can wear them longer without fear of tearing or cracking.

Ridged nails Buffing can help smooth the appearance of ridges but be sure to check out the cause first. Ridging is usually evident after illness or from external trauma to the nails. Strong medication can also cause an uneven nail surface and often they will return to normal once the medication has stopped. Ridge filler is a product that 'fills in' the nail ridges giving a smooth overall appearance so try this and see if it works. Alternatively, buff with a four-way buffer to increase circulation at the base of the nail (matrix) and to smooth the surface of the nails. Do not buff too regularly or too hard as this thins the nails irreparably and will increase the risk of breakages.

Green fungal infections These are very common and are usually caused by unhygienic nail equipment or water becoming trapped under a nail extension! Both can be treated with specific non-prescription anti-fungal nail ointment produced by many nail cosmetics companies. Sanitising your nail kit regularly will ensure infections happen rarely, if at all, and a professional application of artificial nails will prevent water seeping into crevices where it can become stagnant under the nail tip. Try not to buff away the green appearance as this will cause increased damage to the already delicate surface of the nail.

Skin identification

It is just as important to identify your skin type as it is your nail type so you can moisturise and hydrate with a suitable product. Not all heavy creams suit all skin types and some respond much better to a moistening gel or natural water spritz.

Because the skin on our hands and feet is at our body's extremities it is used every day very regularly and always exposed to the environment so the pressure on these areas is immense. Yet most of us rarely use products to protect these areas against nature's ravages.

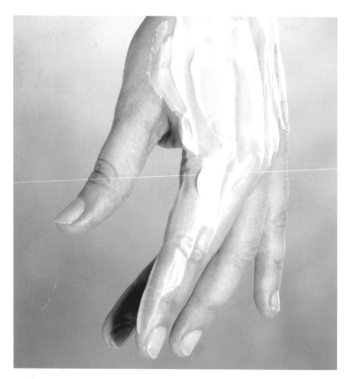

△ *Use oil-based cream preparations on dry skin to secure moisture and delay the onset of the 'mature' look.*

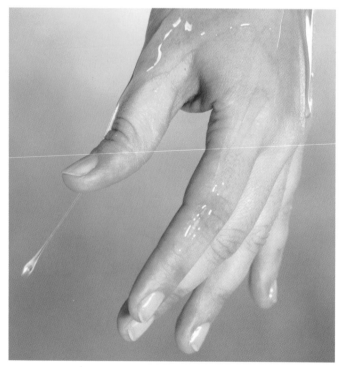

△ *Dehydrated skin needs a boost of water both externally and internally, so make sure you drink lots of water.*

Dry skin More often than not the skin on our hands and feet will be dry and this dryness will need to be treated with an emollient cream rich in oils to provide a barrier against water loss. Hot oil and wax treatments are great for renourishing the skin and helping it become more susceptible to nutritious product ingredients. Dry skin does need regular treatment so carrying a hand cream or foot cream with you is advisable. Try to moisturise after washing hands and feet or when wearing sandals. Cracking of hand and foot skin is painful so prevention is better than cure!

Dehydrated skin Dehydration is caused by a lack of water in the skin due to over use of detergents or bleach in cleaning fluids. A lotion moisturiser will work wonders by replacing lost moisture and removing the dry, dull appearance of the skin in favour of a smooth and silky finish.

Sweaty skin Often nervous tension will make our palms perspire and when meeting new people there is little more off-putting than shaking a wet hand! Regularly apply mattifying cream to the hands to reduce the wetness of the palms and guard the skin against the sodium (salt), found in sweat which can dry the skin and make it flaky. Foot perspiration is another matter altogether and wearing airy shoes helps to circulate fresh, cool air around the feet. Try using foot powder regularly, too, as this will help to absorb the perspiration and at least give a drier feel to the feet.

Ageing skin Skin begins to age from the age of 21 and our hands are no exception. They are also one of the only areas on the body where plastic surgery is virtually impossible so preventing signs of ageing is essential as there is no cure! Ageing of the hands occurs mainly because of the UV rays from the sun which damage the cells that give skin its stretchy, plumped appearance. This degeneration manifests itself as sagging, wrinkly skin, a result that is almost impossible to reverse. However, regular use of hand lotion and some SPF products will prevent further damage occurring. 'Age spots' – large brown moles on the back of the hands – are also caused by sunlight and products are constantly being developed to diminish their appearance.

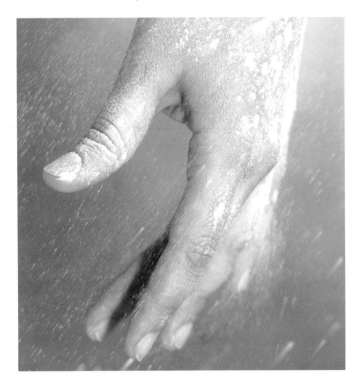

△ Skin that perspires easily can be masked with a light powder or mattifying lotion which absorbs the moisture and maintains softeness.

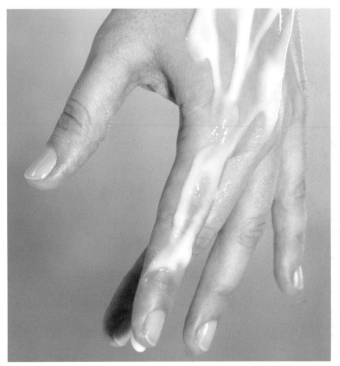

△ Ageing skin on hands and feet loves water and cream- or oil-based products, so daily nourishing is essential.

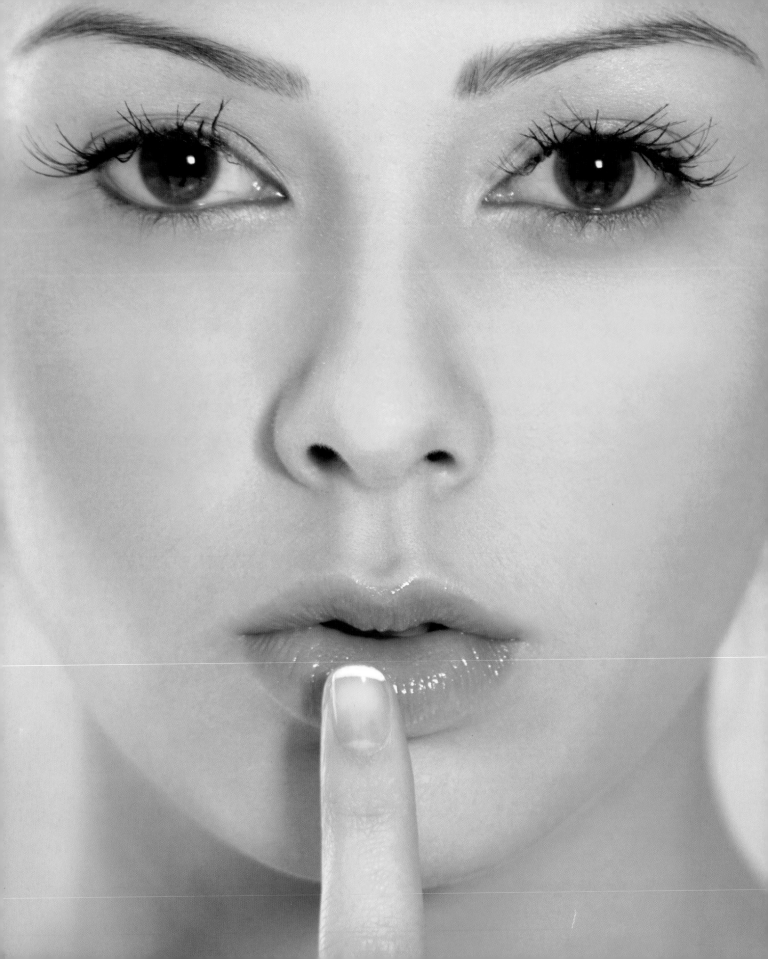

03 the challenges

the challenges

A professional nail technician will be able to identify any nail conditions or changes in the appearance of the nails that suggest that a manicure or pedicure should not be carried out.

These changes are called 'contra-indications' and this simply means a reason not to go ahead with treatment, usually because the risk of cross infection is high or the treatment could be painful. Many nail diseases can also cause unsightly problems but thankfully most of them can be easily treated.

The challenges

Either yourself or a nail technician can successfully treat a number of nail conditions. The following are common conditions that can be easily treated without medication.

Ridges and furrows are simply lines that run along the length of the nail. They can either be superficial or deep lines but the deeper ones are usually caused by illness or strong medications and the superficial lines are caused by external trauma to the nail like banging.

Leuconychia is identified as white spots on the nail plate which are caused by damage to the nail matrix as it grows. It is very common and prevention involves treating the nails more gently! This painless nail bruise is basically a small air pocket which will eventually grow out. There is no treatment but the spots can be covered with coloured varnish.

Hang nails are loose pieces of skin that break away from the nail wall and can be painful if caught and torn. Treat these by using cuticle nippers to remove the skin before it causes infection or pain.

Thickening of the nails is called onychauxis and can occur because of trauma to the toenails due to badly fitting shoes. Treatment involves removing the ill-fitting shoes and buffing the nails to reduce their thickness until they begin to grow normally again.

Onychophagy is the Greek name for very bitten nails! It is a condition were the individual constantly bites and wears down the length of the nail plate, sometimes so severely that there is very little nail left, leaving the nail bed open to bacteria and fungal infections as well as being painful. Try to stop biting the nails by using a 'stop bite' treatment which tastes revolting and will hopefully put you off!

▽ *These nail problems do not prohibit a nail treatment but assess the nails on the day you wish to treat them as they may feel painful.*

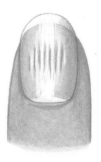
△ Furrows

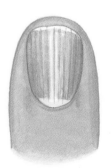
△ Ridges

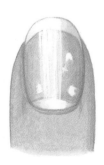
△ Leuconychia

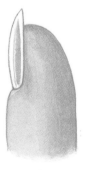
△ Hangnail

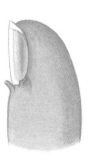
△ Onychauxis

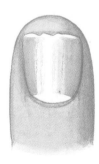
△ Onychophagy

Contagious catastrophies

Some nail problems are in fact diseases and nail treatment is unwise as the risk of spreading the disease to yourself or others is high. The most widespread disease is called tinea unguium and is commonly known as ringworm of the nails. It gives the nails an opaque and dull colour and makes them flaky and rough to the touch. It is caused by a fungal infection of the free edge which transmits itself to the matrix and affects growth. It can be easily medically treated but nail treatments should be avoided at all costs until the disease has been completely eradicated. Equally tinea pedis, or athlete's foot, is also a contra-indication to treatment as it is highly contagious and must be treated with medication before attempting pedicure treatments.

It is also highly unadvisable to treat skin with undiagnosed lumps and bumps. Get these checked out by the doctor first and then carry on with treating yourself. Any cuts or bruises can be painful if treated and broken bones and muscle strains are best left alone until they have healed fully. Warts and skin lesions can be highly infectious so stop the chances of them spreading by not treating your hands or feet until they have cleared.

Some severe types of psoriasis and eczema are very painful and certain nail preparations can make them worse so seek the advice of a medically trained person or a dermatologist before continuing. Always trust your instincts and if you see something which is out of the ordinary get yourself checked out.

Bone conditions

Arthritis usually affects people in older age but there are forms of the disease which affect people of all ages, even children. The cartilage surrounding the ends of bones is degenerated with this condition and so the joints appear swollen and are painful. Some forms of massage can help soothe joint pain but others just aggravate the condition so proceed with care.

Heat treatments such as hot oil and wax treatments are great for these types of sore joints as they increase blood flow without straining any of the surrounding muscles and tendons. Broken and brittle bones are too delicate to treat with massage so take your doctor's advice before attempting these treatments. Gout is another joint inflammation disease and was known as the 'rich man's disease' as it was thought to arise from excessive living and a high consumption of red

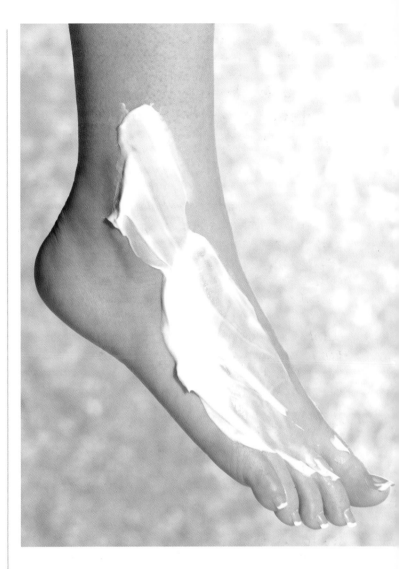

wine and red meat! This is better off being treated by a doctor first and once the painful joints subside, nail and massage treatments can continue.

Bunions are essentially where the toe's joint is thickened and distended due to excess pressure from ill-fitting shoes or extreme weight gain. Reversing the problem is difficult so it is vital to give toes the room they need to grow without hindrance from shoes.

Muscle conditions

There are many muscles in the hands and feet and we use them all the time. Muscle pain and strain is common in these delicate areas and it is inadvisable to massage or treat muscles already under stress or those that have been damaged.

Hands and feet have flexible joints that provide a wide range of movements. However, utilising a few movements repeatedly can cause pain in some areas of the fingers and wrists. Typing and sewing are examples of concentrated movements practised regularly. Repetitive strain injuries (RSIs) like these come in different forms and one group of conditions which affects most of us is that of occupational overuse syndrome. These are a collection of muscle strains, pains and weaknesses which can have long- or short-term effects.

Carpal tunnel syndrome is a painful condition where nerves in the wrist receive too much pressure and subsequently give off a tingling numb sensation. This condition worsens over time and is usually most painful when awakening after sleep. Always consult your doctor and avoid painful movements. Often support bandages are given out until the problem is under control and some medication for pain relief is prescribed. To prevent his condition affecting you change the way you work and your posture regularly to give your muscles and bones the benefit of variety.

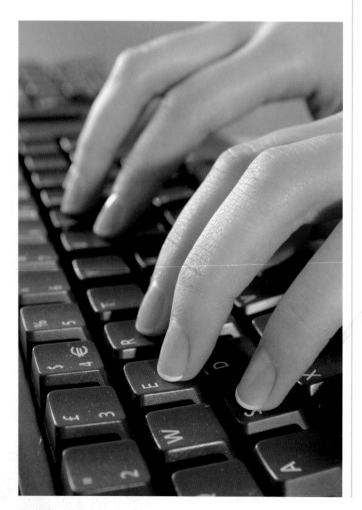

Tenosynovitis and **epicondylitis** are both conditions which affect the tendons of joints and bones in overused areas like the neck, shoulders, wrists and hands. Try to use a range of movements throughout the day, like changing the side your computer mouse is on or holding the phone in a different position. These minor changes can really make a difference.

Nervous conditions can also cause hand and foot problems. Twitching and shaking can be common to some people but not to others so any noticeable changes need to be checked by your doctor.

Nail disorders

Nail disorders are far more serious than nail conditions and they are all best left treated medically to protect non-affected nails from cross infection or contamination. All nail disorders and diseases have Greek- and Latin-derived names like most anatomical study but they can be described easily for identification:

Fungal infections can be caused by many different types of fungus and can be contracted in many ways, from poor hygiene routines to direct contact with the fungus or poor application of false nails. The nail will usually become porous around the infected area and turn a yellowy green colour. If left untreated, the nail will begin to crumble as the keratin is dissolved. There are many treatments for these types of infection. After professional diagnosis has taken place make sure you receive treatment as soon as possible to prevent further damage or other nails becoming infected.

Contact dermatitis is caused by an allergic reaction to a substance or product placed on the skin. Usually jewellery metals can spark a bout of dermatitis but chemicals used in the application of false nails can also be an irritant. The symptoms are a red, inflamed and itchy area which is hot and painful. Treatment initially consists of removing the irritant, whether it be jewellery or the false nails, and then treat the skin with antiseptic substances until it returns to normal.

Haematomas are likely to be suffered by runners and athletes. This is when the nail is banged and a small amount of blood is released and trapped between the nail plate and the nail bed. More often than not the nail will lift from the bed and fall off, however, releasing the pressure built up by the trapped blood can help prevent this action. Often the pain and pressure are released with a small puncture made in the nail plate by a heated pin. This procedure is best carried out by a medical expert to prevent the risk of infection and to ensure that the nail is correctly dressed with a plaster or bandage. Ill fitting shoes can also encourage haematomas so wearing the correct shoes for your feet will go some way to preventing this unsightly occurrence.

Common skin complaints

Some skin disorders like psoriasis and dermatitis can adversely affect the appearance of the nails and consulting a dermatologist is vital to prevent these disorders spreading. Additionally, some foot or hand problems can be brought on by ill-fitting footwear or repeated stress caused by manual jobs.

Calluses and **corns** are common foot complaints but can be treated easily. They are skin complains caused by thickened layers of skin, usually the result of friction or pressure in a particular area. Regular use of a foot file or pumice will diminish their appearance but to truly stamp out the problem footwear must fit correctly and must not rub against the skin.

Blisters too are found on the skin of the feet and these are superficial sacks of liquid which build up to protect the deeper dermal layers of the skin from damage from rubbing shoes. The process of 'breaking in' shoes should not take more than one wear otherwise your feet will suffer and pain could be caused unnecessarily.

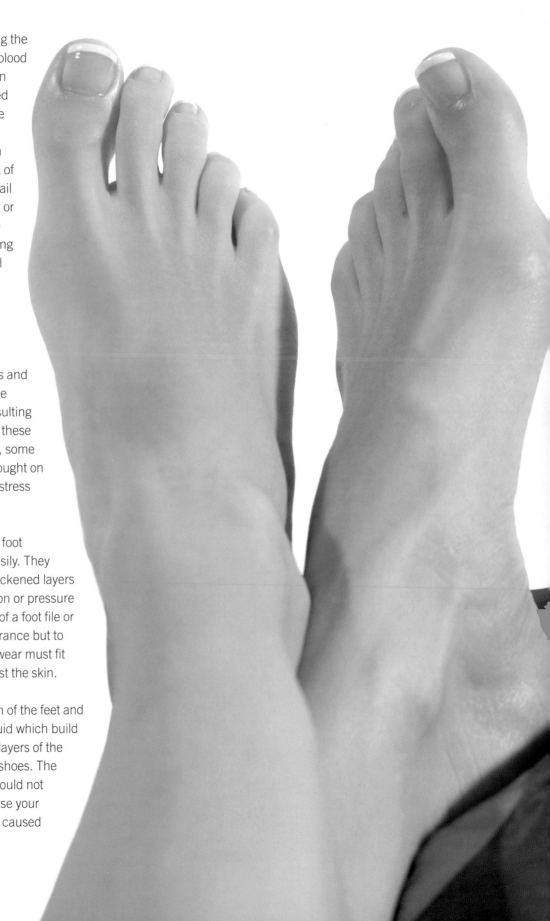

the extreme close-up

In this day of high gloss beauty and fashion there is increasing pressure to look immaculate at all times! The feet and hands are no exception and so one of the first rules not to forget is unwanted hair on toes and fingers...

Waxing

If your feet are on display it is essential that they are free of hair. Even men are now waxing their toes, much to the appreciation of their partners! The elegant look of deep plum coloured toenails will be overshadowed by hairy toes and feet so make sure you invest a little time in a quick and effortless wax!

Waxing should always be done by a professional but if you do decide to try it yourself here are a few golden rules you should follow:

★ If warming the wax in the microwave do not heat it too much and always test it first on the inside of your wrist – burned skin is not a good look!

★ The toes and fingers can be cooler than other hairy areas so make sure you remove the wax as soon as possible to prevent it sticking steadfastly to your skin!

★ Use proper wax! Pre-waxed strips are like sticky tape and will remove more skin than hair!

★ Always apply a cream, gel or oil aftercare to prevent bacteria invading the open hair follicles and to moisture the skin whilst removing the residue of sticky wax.

The pain-free option!

Should you not wish to wax or haven't time to take a trip to your local beauty salon you could try bleaching unwanted hairs to tame their appearance. Thick, dark hair can be unsightly whereas light, bleached hair will be less obvious. Shaving the hair is not a good option as it will grow back very quickly and leave a stubble, so unless you want to shave every time you shower try another method of removing hair, like plucking or threading.

Usually most hair is found on the big toe so a quick pluck here will do the trick for a number of weeks. You may also wish to try hair removal cream but bear in mind it works in a similar way to shaving and lasts about as long, so if you are looking for a long-term fix this is not it.

A more permanent option is epilation or laser therapy to rid toes and fingers of unwanted hair for good. Because the areas treated are small you will find treatment quick and effective but these areas can be very sensitive so be prepared for a little pain.

Botox

Botox is now being used to help people with open foot wounds, such as ulcers. The muscle freezing action of clostridium botulinum bacterium has powers which have not only been a treatment for ageing skin and wrinkles, Tourette's syndrome and muscle spasms but it is also now being used on feet! In the modern day of high-heeled shoes, feet can get sore and painful due to the extreme positions they are

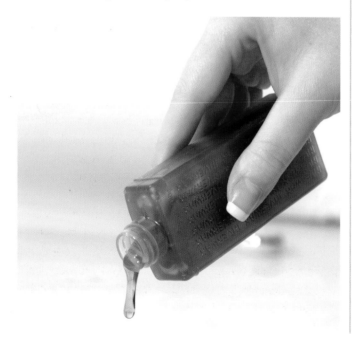

WAXING

Never try to go fast with waxing. Work on one area at a time and apply the wax thinly and in small patches to prevent removal problems. Remember that once on, wax can only come off with a strip so persist but do not wax any area more than twice as the skin will become red and sore.

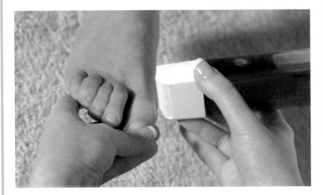

△ Apply the wax to the area being treated in the direction of hair growth.

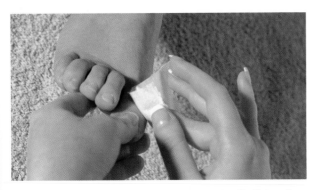

△ Press a muslin trip onto the waxed area and pull off sharply against the hair growth.

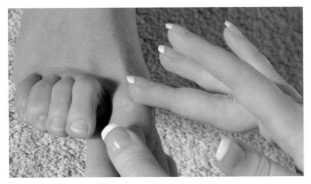

△ Finally, soothe redness and cool the skin with an aloe gel or after-wax oil

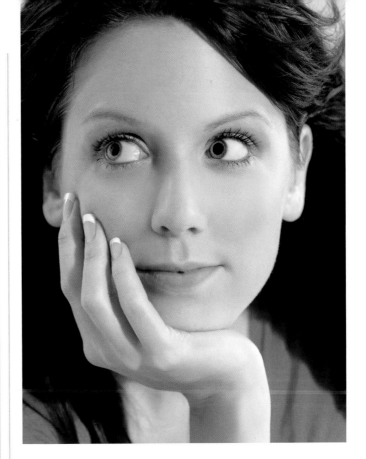

subjected to. Feet are not trained to be regularly hyper extended and so instead of wearing more sensible shoes celebrities are combating foot arch pain with Botox injections.

Attention please!

Most of us are happy with a manicure or pedicure to tidy and spruce the nails but what if you want the main focus of the night to be your feet or hands? These days you can be as outrageous as you like in whichever way you choose to express yourself!

Feet should always be looked after, regardless of the shoes you wear. Some women are very comfortable in stilettos, others in wedges and some in nothing but flats! Whatever works for you is fine but the more unnatural pressure you apply to your feet the more pressure they are under to rebalance your body.

As young children it is vital to allow feet to freely grow and so shoes should never be restrictive or high because as the feet grow the muscles and bones form quickly. If a child wears high shoes the muscular arch under her foot can be stretched unnaturally and so when the shoes are removed the child is unable to return the foot to the ground and walks constantly on her toes!

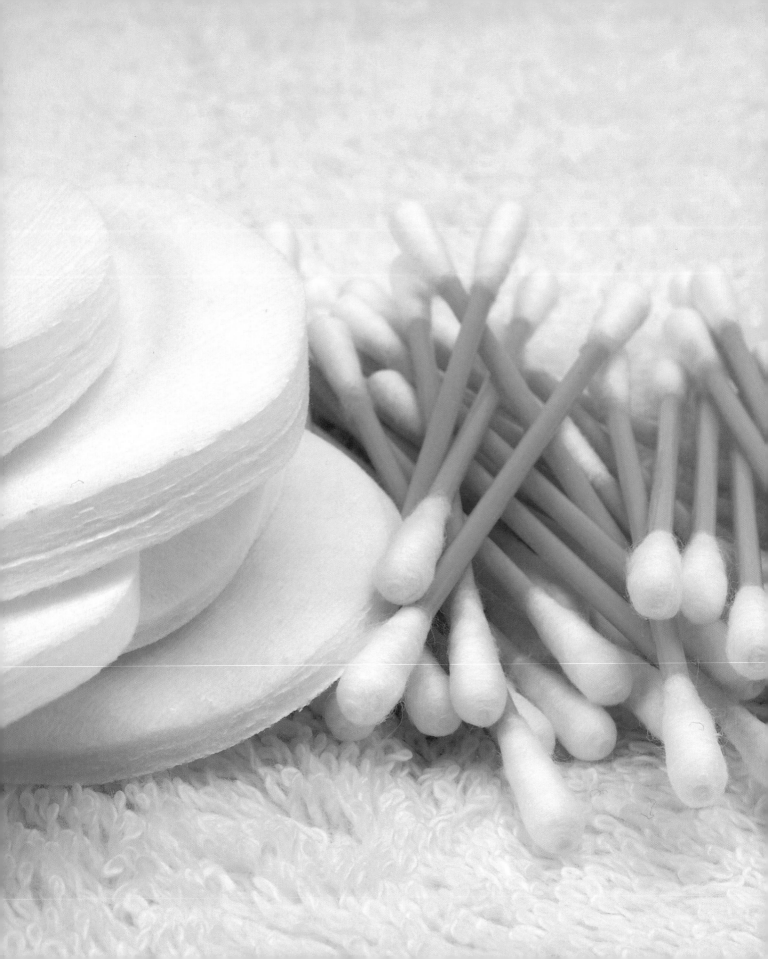

04 the tools

the tools

If you are on the quest for beautiful nails you won't achieve them unless you have the right tools. Nail products and equipment are not cheap but are very worthwhile. Making life easy for yourself will save you time and money in the long run.

Most nail tools are generic and can be used for both manicures and pedicures but some specialised tools are also superb for very specific jobs. Try not to get carried away, however, and don't be tempted to overspend on tools. Be realistic and buy what you can afford. Basic tools nearly always come in kit form and in a handy case so try this to begin with. You can always invest in more specialised equipment to add to your tool box as you become more familiar with what works best for you and your clients.

TOOLS LIST

① Acrylic brushes
② Block buffers
③ Toe separators
④ Acrylic dapendish
⑤ Cuticle knife
⑥ Extension clippers
⑦ Nail clippers
⑧ Nail scissors
⑨ Cuticle nippers
⑩ Orange wood stick
⑪ Sanitiser spray
⑫ Grit nail files
⑬ Nail extension tips
⑭ Nail resin
⑮ Foot rasp
⑯ Acrylic nail 'form'
⑰ Pumice and nail brushes
⑱ Cuticle oil

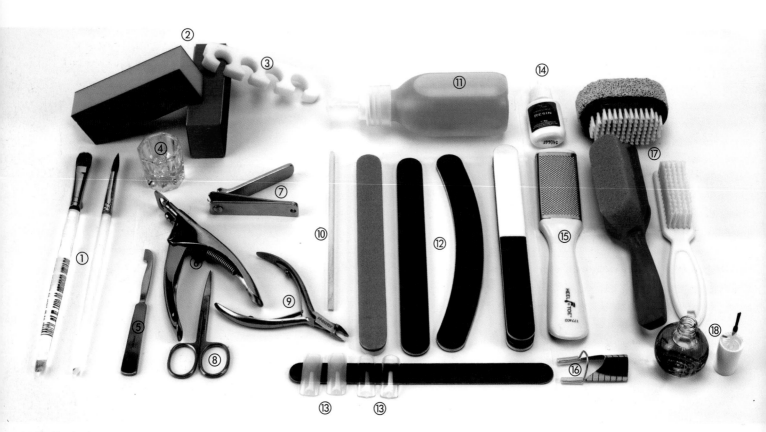

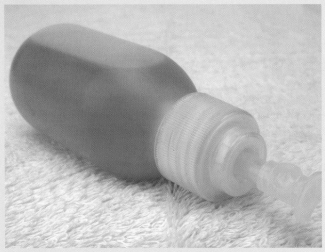

Sanitiser Regular use of sanitiser on yourself and your tools will prevent bacterial and fungal infections spreading. Spray your tools and hands before starting a nail treatment. No reputable nail bar technician will move on to the next client without sterilising all the equipment first.

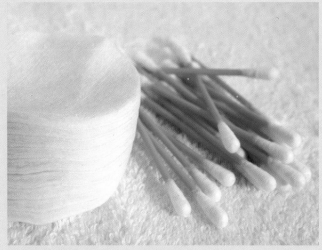

Cotton buds and cotton wool Cotton buds are useful for removing varnish and cleaning cuticles after varnishing. Cotton wool of any variety is simply great for absorbing varnish, liquids and oils so any slips or smudges can be fixed. Always have a good supply to hand!

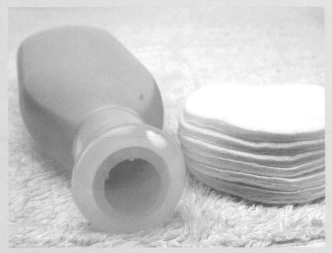

Nail varnish remover Always use an acetone-free remover to clean the nails and remove excess or old polish. Harsh chemicals in other forms of varnish remover do the job faster but dehydrate the nails, making them brittle and dull in appearance. Varnish removing pads and pens are all available for you to try but be sure to test them before you buy as some are just gimmicks, designed to make life easier but actually don't!

Nail soak and bowl During any nail treatment it is vital to soak and cleanse the area being treated after you have removed the risk of infections spreading by using a sanitiser. Use a free-standing bowl for the hands and a pedi spa for the feet but be sure to include a generous squirt of anti-bacterial foam to the water to protect your equipment and cleanse the skin. Aromatherapy oils can also be added to the bowls to give a relaxing twist to the treatment. Nail cleaning agents like fuzz balls and fizzy oxygen-rich bombs can be used to clean under the nails and lighten them whilst cleaning them.

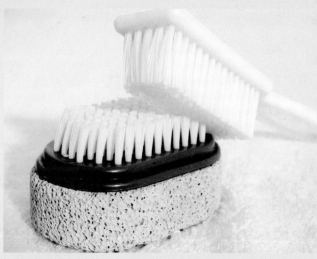

Nail brush This will enable you to really reach underneath the nails' free edge to clean any dirt or grime from beneath them. The brush also helps to remove any oil from the nails when used with water and cleanser so use before the treatment starts and just before varnishing to ensure the nails are squeaky clean!

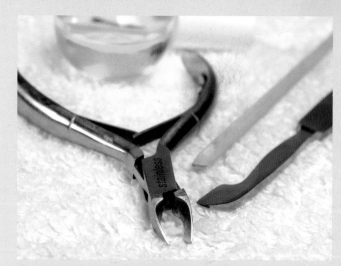

Cuticle equipment Several tools are used to treat the cuticles. The orange wood stick and the hoof stick both serve the purpose of pushing back the cuticles. These can also help lift excess cuticle for removal. Cuticle knives are used to gently remove surface skin cells that may hinder the smooth application of varnish. Use cuticle nippers and blades to cut away excess cuticle and to remove hang nails. Ensuring blades are sharp is essential as the cutting action should be clean and not tear or pull.

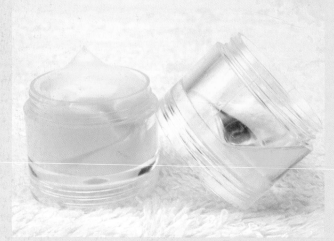

Cuticle treatments Cuticle removers come in liquid form and are usually painted onto the cuticles. Other types of treatment include creams or oils. These should be used regularly to prevent cuticles becoming unruly. Rub into the cuticles, then dip the fingers or toes in warm water for a few minutes. Remove all traces of product as some chemicals found in the bases can carry on working if not rinsed off properly and can make the fingers and nails red and swollen.

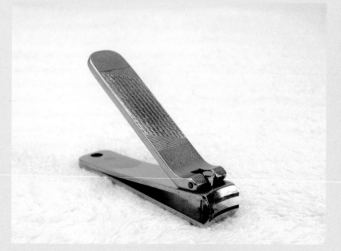

Nail clippers Only ever use to remove length from the nail, and not to shape them. Clippers should always be used instead of scissors as they put less pressure on the sides of the nails, preventing splitting.

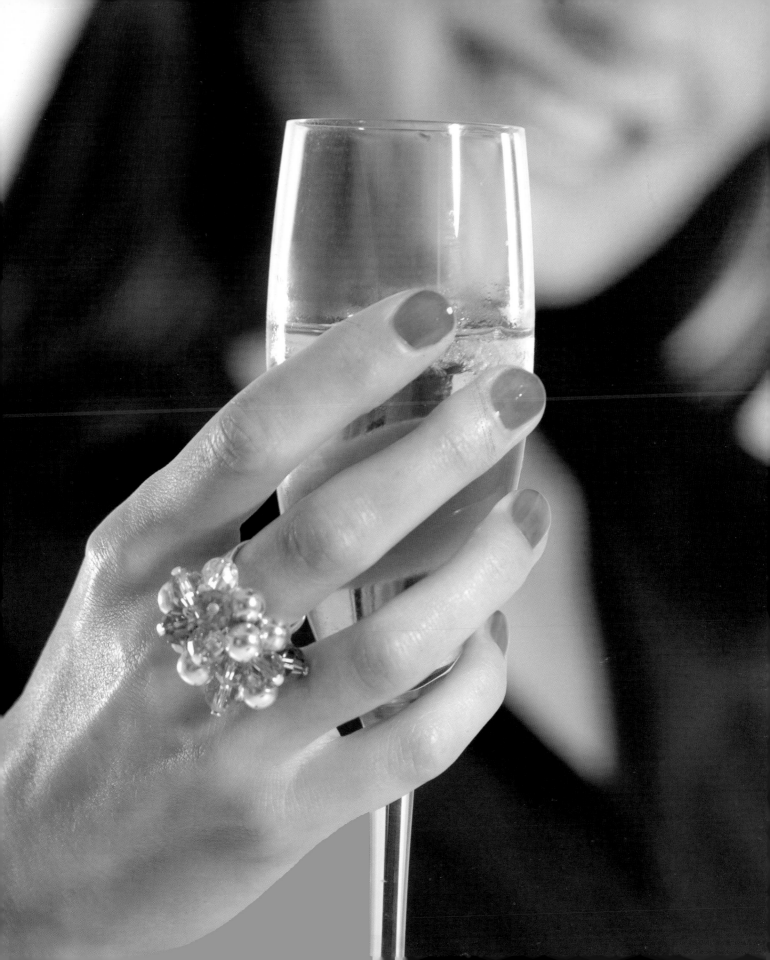

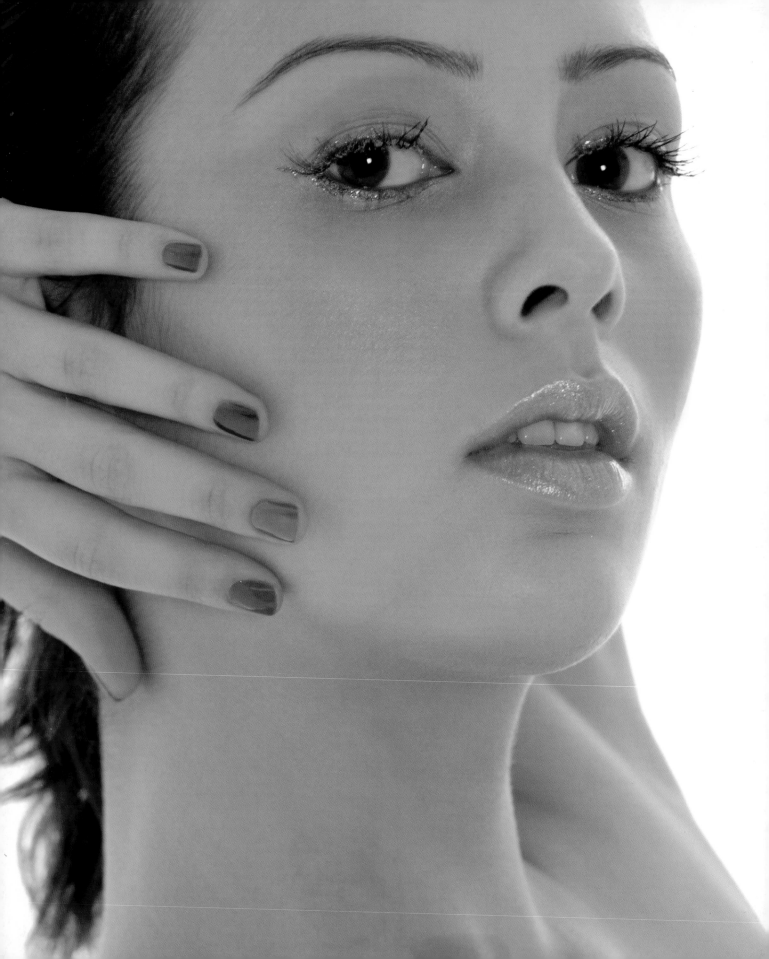

Nail files These come in many forms, shapes and sizes and are no longer just made of paper and metal. Nail files now come in glass, Perspex, gel and fibreglass. The best ones are thin enough to use under the nail but fine enough to remove nail slowly and not to take too much away in one fell swoop! Nail files are graded by numbers which indicate how gritty their surfaces are – the heavier the grit the quicker the nail will be filed away. A classic nail emery board can be too sharp for thin or weak nails but also too fine for toenails so have a board for your fingernails and one for your toenails. Two-sided files are often even better as one side will be gritty enough to take the length off the nails while the other side is used to smooth the edges. Avoid metal files as they are too harsh on the nail without effectively removing the length you wish.

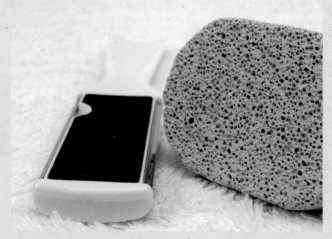

Skin files, rasps and pumice stones These skin removers are excellent on feet and are best used lightly and after a warm soak. There are many types of foot files and these can be metal, paper, wooden, pumice stone or glass but the best offer both a harsh removal element and a buffing smoothing effect.

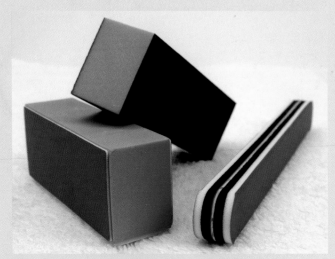

Nail buffers Use these sparingly. A board buffer with various sides is good for general use whereas a block buffer is best used occasionally. Buffing eliminates ridges and shines the nails. Never buff nails more than once a week as this will irreparably thin them and cause the matrix damage. A cream grit buffing paste can be used instead but it is messy and small grit particles can stay on the nail plate and affect the smoothness of the varnish application.

SIMPLE SOLUTIONS FOR PROBLEM NAILS

- For weak, damaged and fine nails use a very fine grit board which allows for a smooth but light removal of nail and a clean shape. Filing may take longer but it will protect your nails against the harsh grit which could tear weak nails.

- For brittle nails, use a medium to heavily grit file as the nail will respond to this much quicker and more effectively.

- For dry nails, use a light to medium file. Dry nails can be worn down quickly by files so go slowly and keep an eye on how much you are removing.

- Nail extensions and very thick nails require around 100/180 grit to effectively smooth them but go slow to avoid damaging the nail plate.

Massage creams and lotions Pampering paradise is all about the massage! Using a rich hand or foot cream will feel luxurious as well as helping to replace lost moisture from the skin and nails. Regular use will promote age-defying hands and feet and make skin feel soft and smooth. If you suffer from excessive sweating of the hands or feet try using a water-based lotion to replace lost moisture whilst protecting the skin from salt found in perspiration lying on the skin. Petroleum jelly does not moisturise the hands, it is just a barrier gel, so if you have dry, cracked hands use a rich oily cream, but not Vaseline, as this does nothing for replacing moisture. Sleeping in hand cream and gloves can aid the extended absorption of creams and lotions but the skin will only absorb so much before it has had enough so after the first 15 minutes there will be very little more absorbed regardless of how long you keep the cream on for!

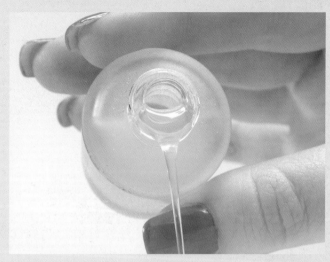

Base coat Base coat is used for two reasons: one is to protect the nails from permanent staining from colour pigments found in varnish and the other is to treat the nails using specific ingredients for a particular nail type. Base coat is vital also for smoothing the nails prior to varnish application and to give extra thickness and protection to the nails. Do not omit base coat as this grass roots stage of varnishing is often the most important.

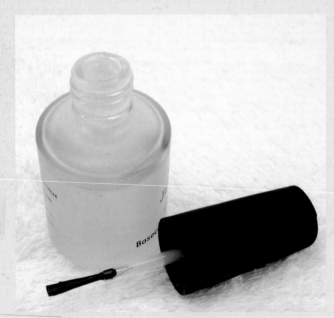

Top coat This is usually used to gloss the surface of nail varnish and to add another layer of protection to the colour. Mattifying top coats for men are now available which coat the nails in protection but offer no nutrient or treatment value.

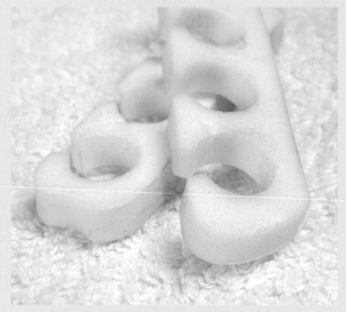

Toe separators These are great for keeping freshly varnished toes apart whilst drying and prevent nail varnish from smudging onto other toes. They are made of sponge and to maintain hygiene keep separators for your toes only!

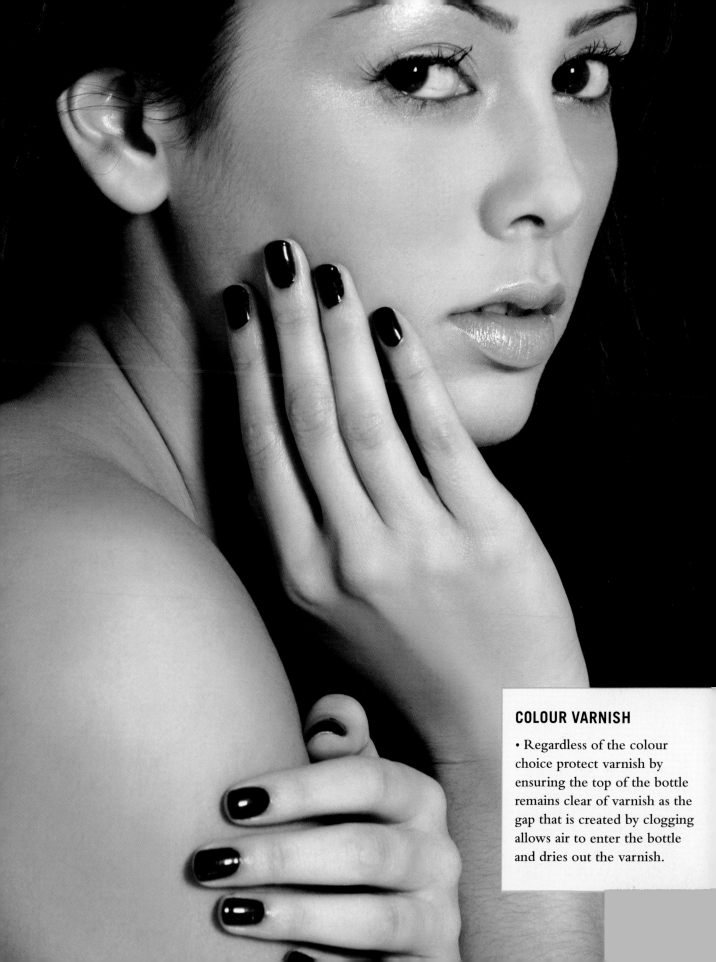

COLOUR VARNISH

• Regardless of the colour choice protect varnish by ensuring the top of the bottle remains clear of varnish as the gap that is created by clogging allows air to enter the bottle and dries out the varnish.

Nail extension equipment

Nail extensions have another set of specific tools which are vital to create a realistic and professional finish to fibreglass, gel and acrylic nails. Regardless of which nail extension system you choose it is important to source the best, most durable products. Recommendations and endorsements are the best ways of surveying the market and often prove to be the best choices. All extension tools tend to be priced similarly so even branded tools won't cost that much more. Using incorrect tools for the job will not create a professional look so invest well and wisely. Whether it be fibreglass, gel, silk or acrylic choose a system that suits you and has the correct look and lasting power!

TOOLS LIST

① Boomerang 100/180 grit file
② Acrylic dapendish
③ Resin activator spray
④ Acrylic liquid base
⑤ Acrylic powders
⑥ Extension clippers
⑦ Nail glue
⑧ Acrylic nail form
⑨ 100/180 grit file
⑩ Nail block buffers
⑪ Acrylic and gel brushes

▽ *Tools of the trade are not only important, they're essential!*

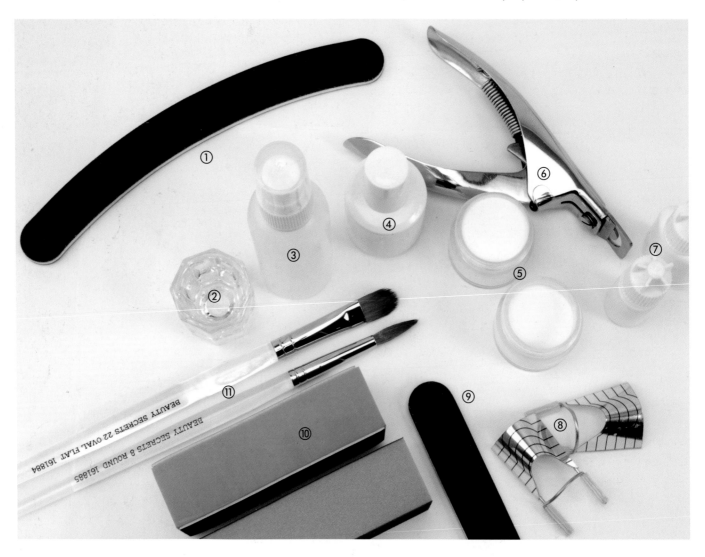

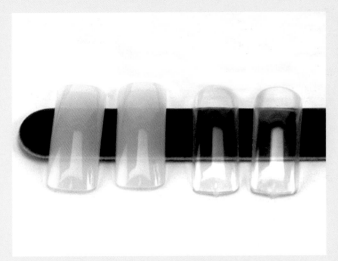

Nail tips These usually come in finger-made sizes and can either be plain or French (white) tipped. Choose the style you wish and cut to size with nail clippers or file down with a nail file. The flexibility of these nails will not affect the end result, however, very hard tips can be prone to shattering so opt for ones that allow movement. Tips are just used to add length to your original nail but fitting them correctly is vital to create the right look so do this carefully.

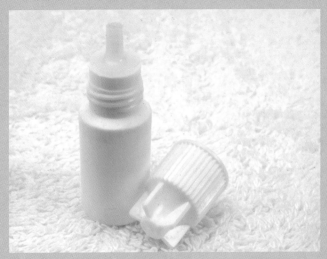

Nail glue Be sure to use the correct nail glue and follow the manufacturer's instructions. Instant glue or super glue will not do and simply isn't strong enough. Pool the glue just on the edge of the tip for the best application.

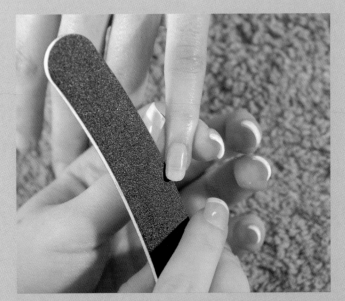

Nail extension files Theses heavy grit buffers come in many abrasive strengths; 100–180 grit is about right for filing acrylic whereas 120–150 is better for the more delicate gel and fibreglass nails.

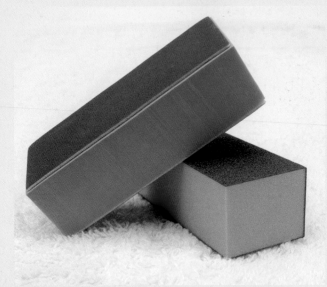

Buffers Buffers should always be blocks and should have different sides to polish and refine the nails. Buffers are used last on unvarnished nails to really smooth the surface of the nails so a very fine grit is needed. The end result should produce a soft shiny surface without ridges or visible lines.

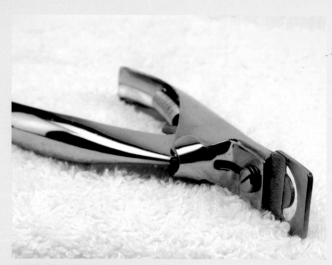

Extension nippers These extension cutters are great for cutting length from extensions without shattering the plastic. Use them at a 90 degree angle for the best edge. Nail scissors or ordinary clippers are not good enough and will shatter the plastic bonding of the extensions, weakening their adherence to the natural nail.

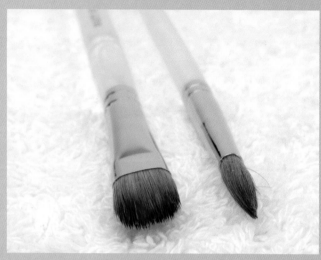

Acrylic brushes Choose a brush that is around size 20–22. It may look big but it will help with the application of acrylic powder in the long run.

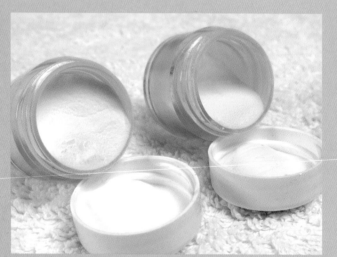

Acrylic powders These fine powders come in clear, French pink and white and are used with acrylic liquid to bond and form the hard coating of acrylic nails. The powder and liquid must not be mixed ahead of time as it hardens and becomes unusable – just mix a little at a time when you are ready to apply.

Acetone Pure acetone liquefies acrylic and nail glue so always have some to hand in case of accidents or if you need to soak the existing nails off. This is a strong substance so do not leave it open as the fumes can give off a potent smell which can spark headaches and nausea. Do not get the liquid into the eyes and if you do, seek medical attention immediately.

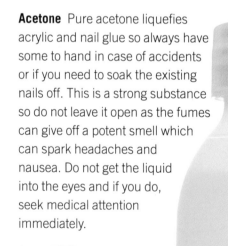

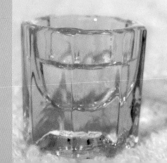

Nail varnishes

Undoubtedly the main reason for having a nail treatment is to make nails look cleaner and well maintained. Regardless of the condition of your nails a varnish, even clear, will boost the overall appearance of the nail plate and make nails look great!

Varnishes come in many colours and some are very expensive. The reason for this is simple: marketing will increase a product's selling power but will also add pounds to its price! Some varnishes are genuinely better than others but price is not a guide. The trick with varnish is not to be sold on the fact that it contains natural vitamins and minerals as they will be ineffective on a dead cell base of nails!

Colour is usually the main pull when buying a varnish and sometimes the brush too can either put you off or encourage a purchase. Check the consistency of the varnish by seeing how it moves in the bottle; varnish that is too thick will simply last half the time of a thinner one. Some of the best known brands are also known to go 'gloopy' very quickly so this test will help make up your mind. Small silver balls are put in varnish bottles to keep the liquidity of its contents and to prevent thickening.

To make coloured varnishes, acrylic polymers are dissolved in solvents and colour pigment added. Nylon or plastics are added to give the varnish flexibility to prevent cracking. Film formers allow the varnish to be applied smoothly and increase adhesion to the nail plate. Formaldehyde is also found in varnishes and this is the main allergy ingredient for nail preparations.

Vigorously shaking the varnish in the bottle creates small air bubbles and spoils the finished result. Instead, simply roll the bottle from side to side to mix the product and let the balls do their magic! Applying coats too soon on top of one another also spoils the smooth finish of varnish. Make sure you allow each coat to dry before applying the next.

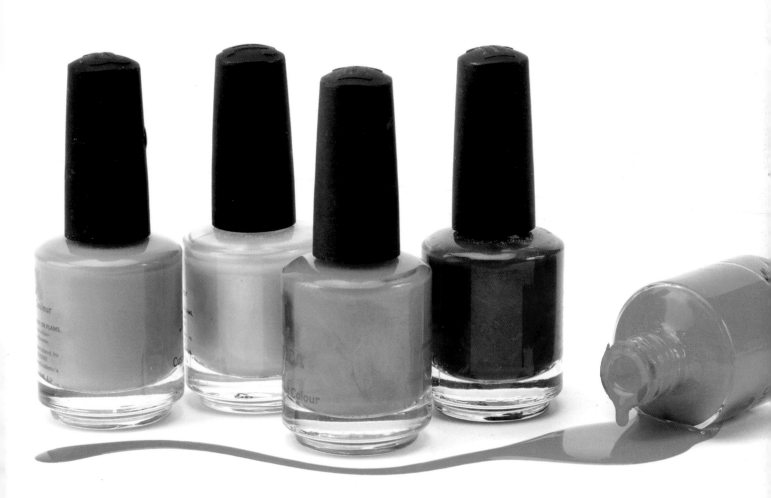

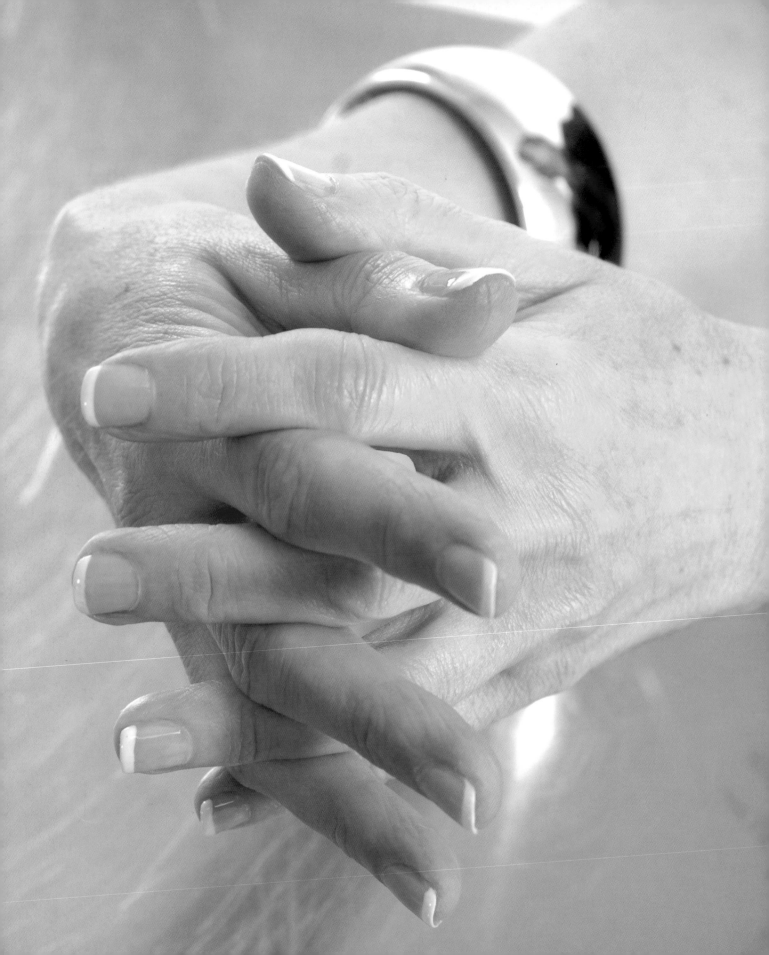

anti-mature

anti-mature

As we grow older our hands and feet show the relentless pressure they have been under over the years. It is virtually impossible to carry out plastic surgery to the backs of the hands and tops of the feet without leaving unsightly scars, so these areas of the body tend to give away our age.

The skin starts ageing from the age of 21 so we must protect the hands and feet from harsh chemicals, overwork and harmful UV rays, all of which accelerate the ageing process. By looking after the hands and feet we can extend their youthful appearance by years.

Toxin block

The environment and over exposure to the sun strip the skin of its youthful collagen and elastin which keep skin looking plump and smooth. Using a sun block on the backs of the hands provides a barrier against all airborne pollutants as well as blocking out UV light which contributes to diminished collagen production as well as unsightly moles and sun spots, all of which are classic signs of aged hands. You need not follow the same daily routine on feet but when they are exposed to the sun it is advisable to provide them with some protection, especially as the skin in this area is usually hidden and the chances of sunburn therefore trebled. Burnt feet are painful as well as unattractive!

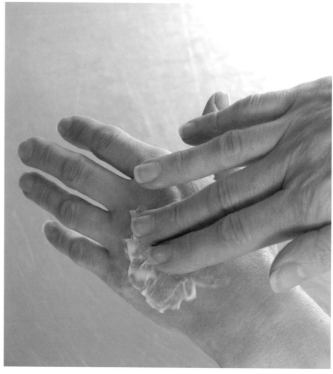

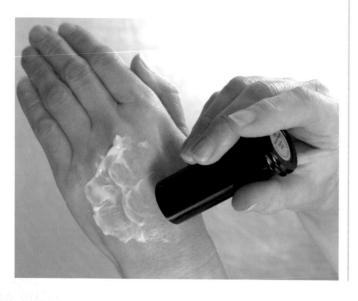

Nourish, nourish, nourish

As the hands and feet age the skin and nails dry in texture and can lack lustre. Maintaining moisture levels is essential to slow this drying process and to keep hands and feet looking and feeling soft and smooth. A light but absorbent moisturising cream for daytime use is ideal as it won't come off on your socks or anything you touch. Thicker creams are great at night because they have all night to sink in. Wearing gloves or plastic bags on your hands won't increase the absorbency of the cream as the very top layers of the epidermis will only absorb as much as they need, softening dead skin cells. So regular applications are more effective.

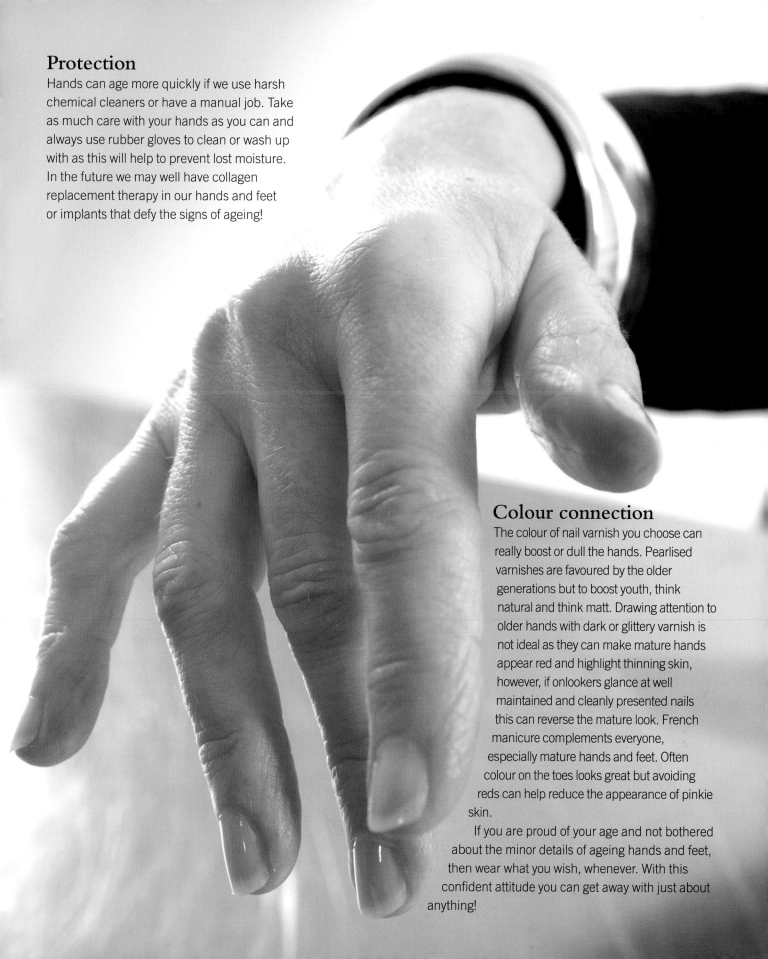

Protection

Hands can age more quickly if we use harsh chemical cleaners or have a manual job. Take as much care with your hands as you can and always use rubber gloves to clean or wash up with as this will help to prevent lost moisture. In the future we may well have collagen replacement therapy in our hands and feet or implants that defy the signs of ageing!

Colour connection

The colour of nail varnish you choose can really boost or dull the hands. Pearlised varnishes are favoured by the older generations but to boost youth, think natural and think matt. Drawing attention to older hands with dark or glittery varnish is not ideal as they can make mature hands appear red and highlight thinning skin, however, if onlookers glance at well maintained and cleanly presented nails this can reverse the mature look. French manicure complements everyone, especially mature hands and feet. Often colour on the toes looks great but avoiding reds can help reduce the appearance of pinkie skin.

If you are proud of your age and not bothered about the minor details of ageing hands and feet, then wear what you wish, whenever. With this confident attitude you can get away with just about anything!

JOINT RELEASE

It is essential to look after older hands and to stretch the joints, releasing tension, muscle pain and possible stiffening of the bones and cartilage. Massage is a great treat you can apply yourself to help mobilise joints and smooth the skin, enabling a greater range of movements and a brighter appearance to the skin. The following exercises can also be carried out on feet. Try a short massage routine every other day to really make a difference.

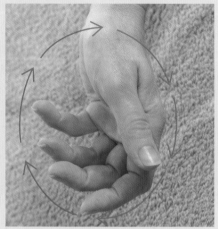

① Start by lightly and slowly circling your wrists to stretch the joint muscles and warm the muscles in the wrist.

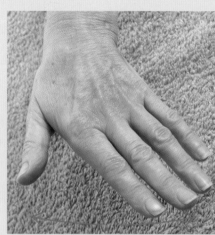

② Next, practise a waving movement from side to side.

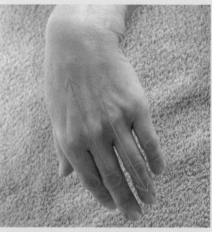

③ Then extend the wave up and down to relax the flexors and extenders of the wrist and lower arm.

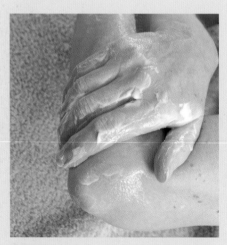

④ Apply cream or oil to the hands and rub them together to warm the medium. Massage up the forearm to the elbow and apply a generous amount of cream or oil to the elbow as this area can get very dry.

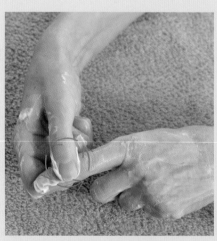

⑤ Apply small circular movements down each finger from tip to base and give each finger a slight pull to finish.

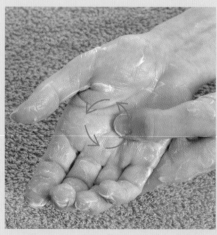

⑥ Massage the palm of each hand with your opposite thumb to relax the muscles of the hands. Finally shake the hands to wake them up, then soak in a warm hand spa.

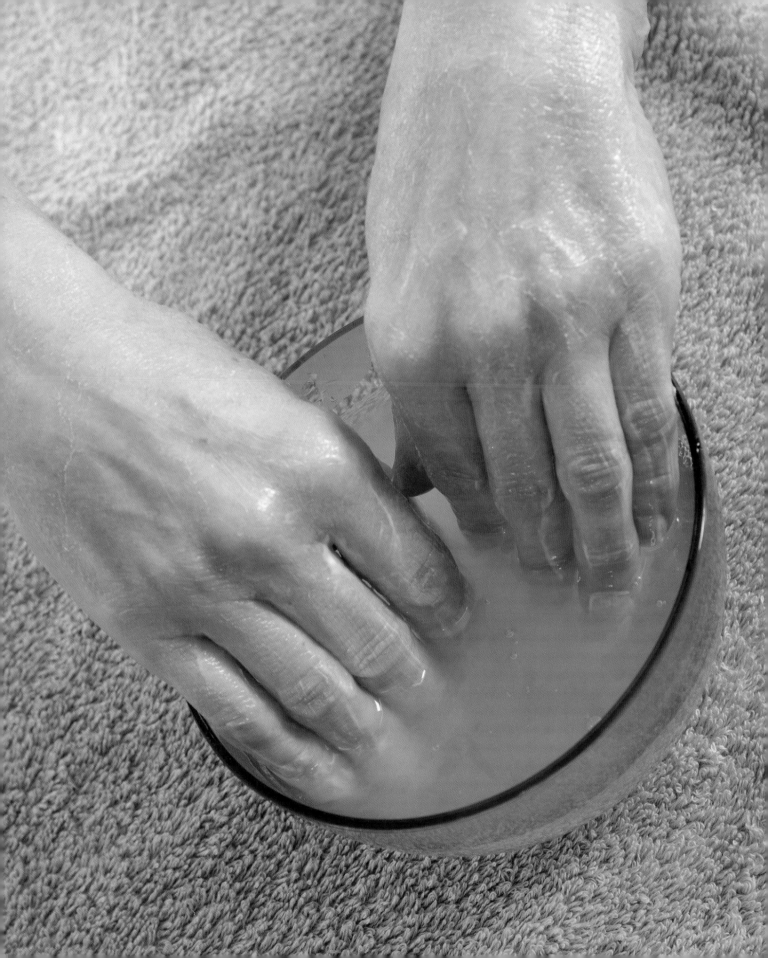

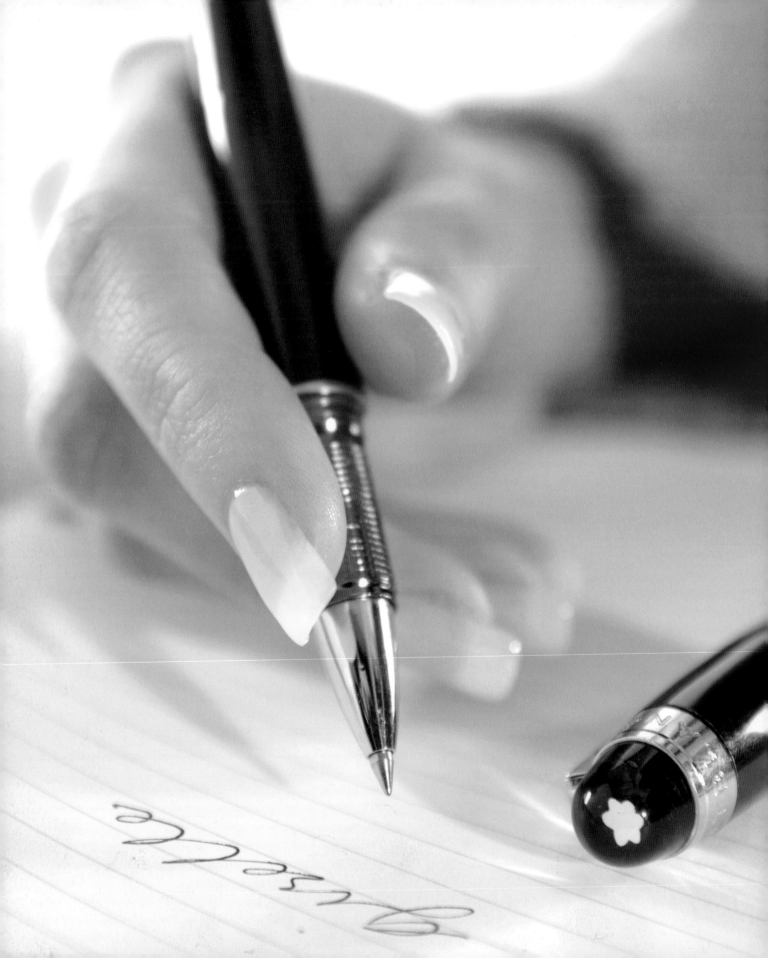

06 the manicure

the manicure

For both men and women achieving fabulous looking groomed nails is really satisfying. A well groomed appearance can make a great first impression and elevate your status! Setting aside a little time to have your nails done regularly and taking pride in your appearance are very positive steps that won't go unnoticed.

Making nails look good takes 20 minutes every week with another 10 minutes added for varnishing so finding the time shouldn't be a problem. There is no excuse! A good manicure with varnish will last seven to 10 days, possibly a little longer if the varnish is hard-wearing and you are doing little with your hands. Top-up treatments can be done at home and consist of regularly moisturising hands and cuticles and filling out any chips.

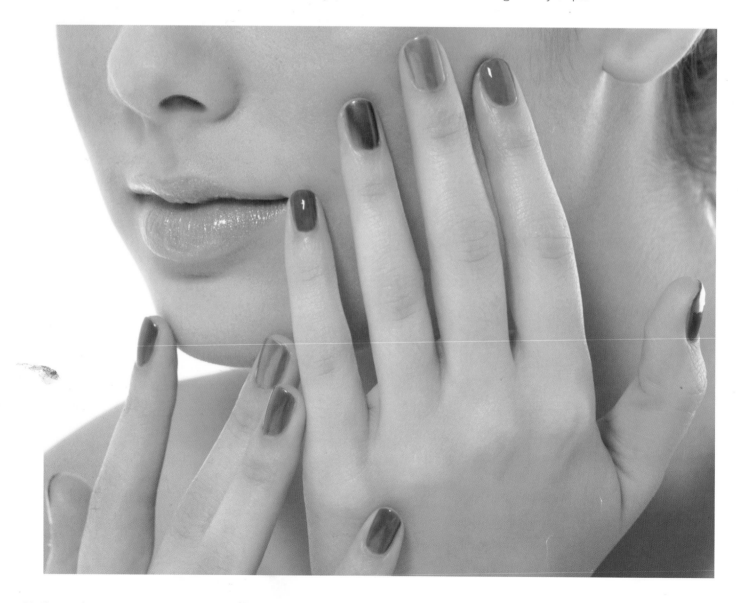

how to...

THE HOME MANICURE

Performing your own manicure at home saves time and money, and is relaxing and satisfying. Treat yourself to 20 minutes of me time once a week and indulge in some self-pampering. Follow the step by steps below and take your time to get them right – it will be worth it in the long run as your nails will look and feel fabulous.

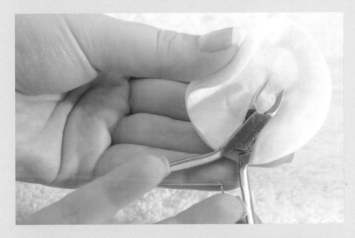

① Ensure your tools are clean and sterilised by wiping them with an antiseptic solution or spraying them with sanitiser. Place them on a clean towel, then wash and dry your hands thoroughly.

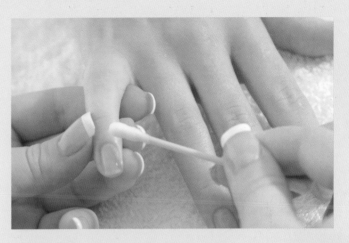

② If the nails are already painted, dampen a cotton wool pad with acetone-free nail varnish remover and remove the old colour. If the varnish is not completely removed, dip a cotton bud into varnish remover and use it to remove excess varnish.

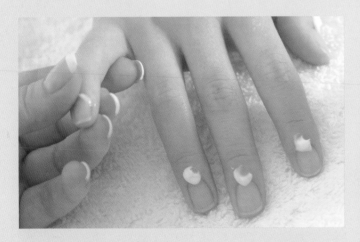

③ Apply a small dot of cuticle remover or cream to the cuticles and rub in. At this stage the cuticles will be hard so it is essential to soften them before manipulating or removing them.

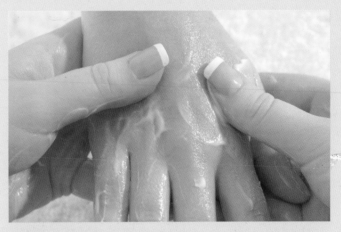

④ Whilst the cream is sinking in, perform a hand and arm massage, using enough massage cream or oil to cover the area. Use any massage routine you like, however, following the routine on pages 64–65 will make sure you stimulate the muscles, bones and blood circulation of the hands and arms.

MASSAGE ROUTINE

Massage has a powerful healing effect on the skin. As well as helping oils to penetrate the skin to nourish it and backtrack the ageing process, massage also helps to alleviate joint strains and pains and increase blood circulation to the tips of the fingers.

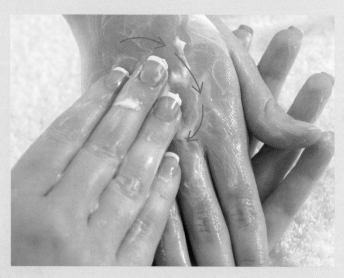

① Apply cream or oil to the hands, then rub them together to increase the intensity of warmth. This warms the oil or cream you are using to help increase slip as well as warming the skin and muscles before the treatment.

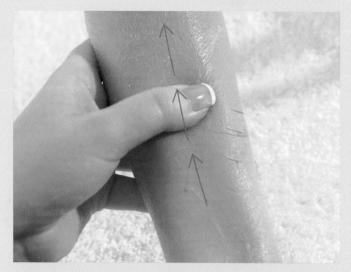

② Knead your forearm with upward movements towards the elbow six times. Remember to work around the two main bones in the lower arm, the radius and ulna, as this feels very soothing. Repeat on the other arm.

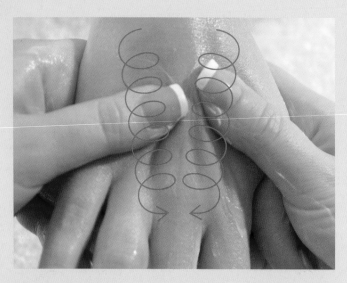

③ Using the thumbs massage in small circles down the middle of the metacarpal bones towards the fingers, then down the fingers. Apply a little pressure to the tips of each finger.

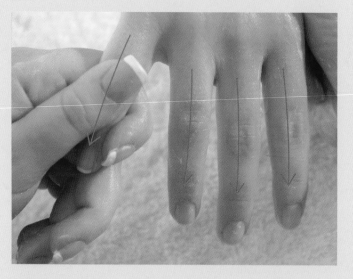

④ Next, alternately pull the fingers away from the hand and slowly release. Complete this movement on all 10 fingers.

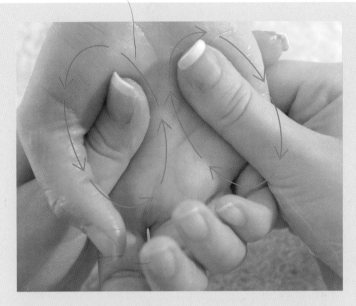

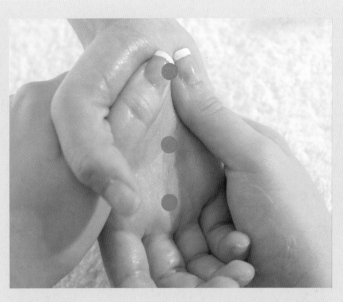

⑤ Turn the hand over and rub the palm in large circles covering the whole area. Deep, slow movements are best all round but pressure is good anywhere on the palm as this is where we find the reflex points.

⑥ Now apply three pressure points to the palm in a line down the centre of the hand. These should be firm and each one should be applied for six second. Taking deep breaths whilst this process is being practised is a great stress reliever.

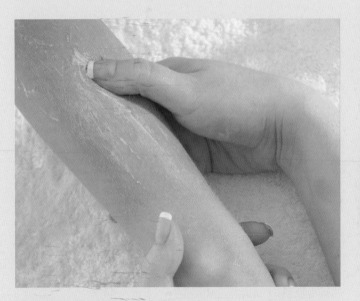

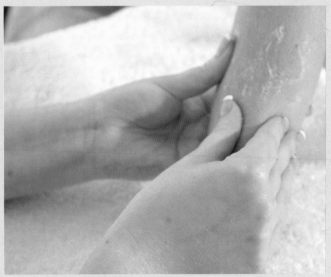

⑦ Next, lightly massage a big circle around the inside of each wrist and follow the same circular action up the arms to the elbows.

⑧ Finally, turn the hand over so the back is facing you and repeat the kneading movements from Step 2 up the hands and arms six times on each arm. Your hands and arms should be slightly pinker than when you started as the blood circulation and muscles have been stimulated. Sometimes a feeling of lightness can occur which is great and proves the massage has worked!

how to...

EXFOLIATION

Exfoliating the hands is best practised after massag as the stimulation to the skin from the massage helps to desquamate the skin twice as effectively. Exfoliating improves the skin's appearance as well as the health of nails.

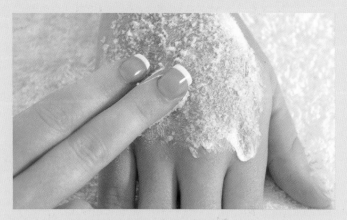

① Exfoliating helps to remove the surface layers of the epidermis through a process of 'desquamation' (peeling). Also, the massage oil or cream will help the small particles of exfoliator slide over the surface of the skin whilst protecting it from harsh particles. Use either a brush or a scrub for this and the smaller the spheres the better as they accomplish the job without damaging the skin's surface. Massage the scrub into the hands and arms, then rinse off.

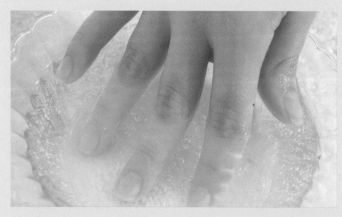

② After a thorough exfoliation, rinse and soak the nails in a bowl of warm water for 5 minutes to soften the cuticles before work on them begins. Pat dry.

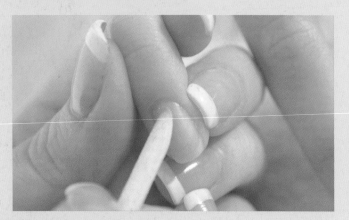

③ Use an orange wood stick to gently push back the cuticles towards the matrix. Be sure also to work along the nail wall as cuticles can grow on the sides of the nail plate, too.

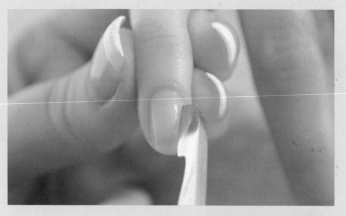

④ Using the cuticle knife, place the blade at a 45 degree slant on the nail and begin to apply small, light circles to the nail plate working from the right nail wall down onto the pushed back cuticle and up the left nail wall side. This should raise and exaggerate any cuticle cells lying on the surface of the plate.

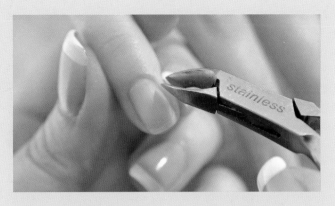

⑤ **To complete the cuticle work, remove any excess cuticles with the nippers. Always be sure to leave some as protection for the matrix.**

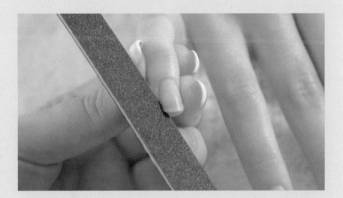

⑥ **Whilst the nails are still a little soft, file them to reduce length and shape the free edge. It is vital not to file a dry nail as too much of the nail's surface can be removed.**

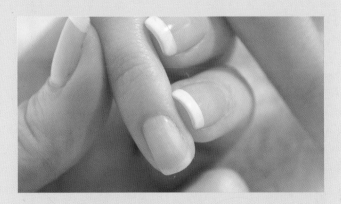

⑦ **Shaping the nails should now be easy but the decision to go square, round or oval may not be!**

Nail shapes

Fashions come and go and nail shapes are no exception! Square or sqoval nails (nails with a tip in between square and oval) are currently in fashion but the best nail shape is one that suits your nails and helps strengthen them. Look at the shape of your cuticle – usually your natural nail shape will mirror this shape to give the most strength. However, well groomed nails suit any shape and will be less likely to break due to the care you have given them.

Squoval nails are also a popular nail shape choice and are still part of the square family with the main difference being the corners of the square nail are filed round.

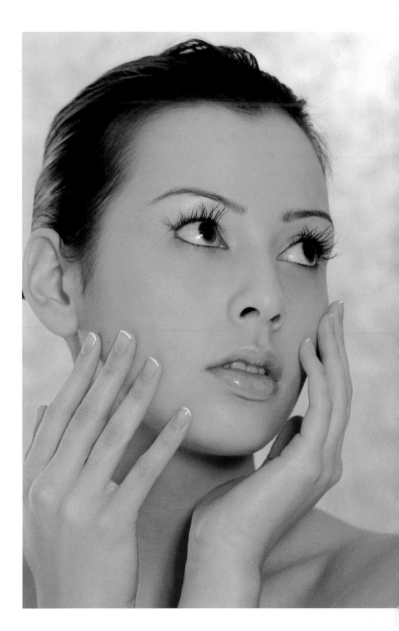

how to...

ROUND NAILS

Round nails are popular with those who prefer a groomed rather than fashionable appearance to their nails. It is better if the nails have some strength to them already as this shape does have weak areas where the nail can split easily.

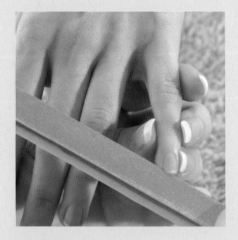

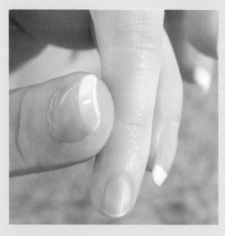

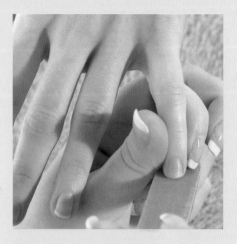

① Working from the side of the nail wall towards the centre, sweep the nail file over the free edge to achieve a round edge.

② As you file check both sides are even by looking at the nail from above and below the fingers.

③ Bevel down the nail to remove any fuzzy edges as this will ensure the varnish lies smoothly and the edge of the nail is not rough or jagged.

OVAL NAILS

This shape was the height of fashion in the 1960s but nowadays not many people opt for this shape as it makes the nails very weak and susceptible to breaks.

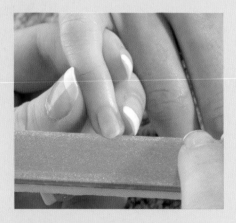

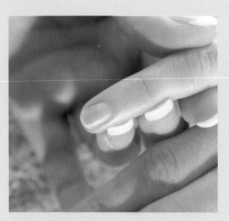

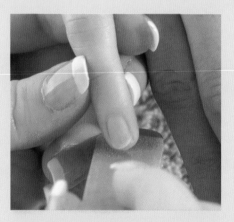

① Following the guidelines for round nails, apply the same technique but file more of the free edge away.

② Do not file away the tip of the nail as the more length left the better but reduce the sides of the nails until the nail is at a rounded point.

③ Bevel as usual to remove fuzzy edges but be careful not to change the shape of the nail at this stage as it is easy to remove too much.

SQUARE NAILS

Square nails are very fashionable especially with French manicure varnish. This shape nail provides extra strength as there are no weak spots. File in one direction only and follow the guidelines below.

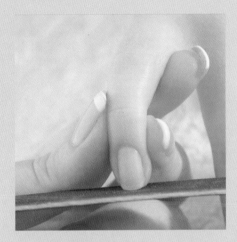

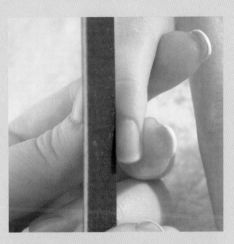

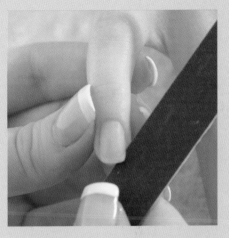

① **Look at the nail straight on and file the free edge down so it is straight across, leaving a 90 degree corner at each side.**

② **Filing in one direction from the side of the free edge to the centre of the nail, file at a 90 degree angle up the nail wall. Very little of the nail should be removed.**

③ **Finally, slightly round off the sides of the nail and, turning the nail file so that it faces down the nail, bevel the nail to remove any fuzzy edges.**

BUFFING

The last phase of the manicure before applying varnish is buffing. This ensures the nails' surface is smooth, shiny and free of oil or creams which could encourage the varnish to lift and chip after application.

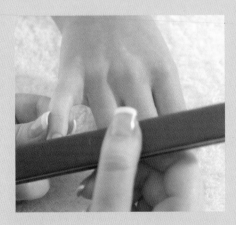

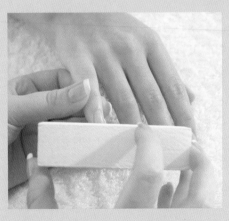

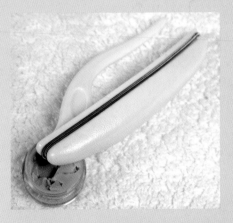

① **The four-way buffer is great on ridges as its various surfaces used in order of roughness (roughest first, smoothest last) treats the nails on a deeper level.**

② **Block buffers are also good for ridges but because they only have one side they will inevitably leave the nails dull so varnish is needed.**

③ **Buffing paste and shammy are good for natural nail wearers as they will buff without removing ridges and simply add shine to the nails' surface.**

how to...

VARNISHING

Varnishing will be difficult to master, especially when varnishing your stronger writing hand with your weaker hand, but persist and the results will pay off. Choose a colour that suits you and ensure the bottle is rolled and not shaken (to avoid the build-up of air bubbles) to thin the varnish before application.

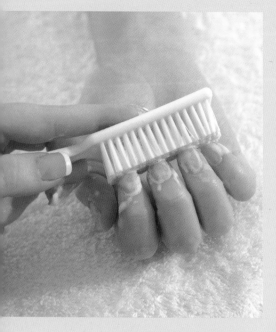

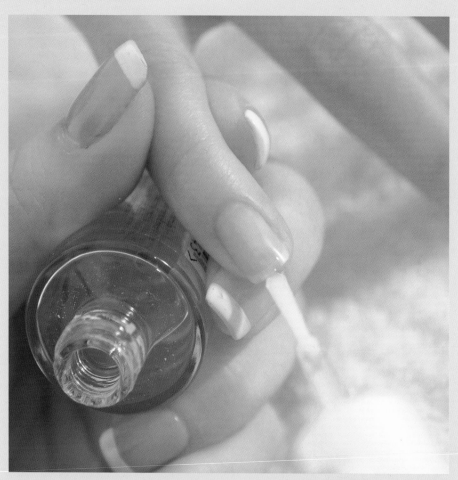

① Before applying varnish, a wet nail brush passed under the free edge will help remove any unwanted debris, such as excess cream or filing dust. Once brushed, pat the nails dry with a towel or paper tissue. Often a tissue or cotton bud run under the free edge will help dry the more difficult to reach areas.

② The varnish is next and if you wish to remain nude, do so! However, a little base coat in a clear colour is best for maintaining shine and adding a layer of protection to the nails' surface. Choose a base coat that treats the nails; you may wish to purchase one that adds moisture, strength or prevents brittle nails shattering. Ensure the base coat also gives protection from the pigment in coloured nail varnish: it is this pigment that makes nails turn yellow! If you are not wearing a colour apply two coats of varnish to give a glossy finish and double the protection; if you are applying colour, apply just one coat of base and then colour on top – the barrier of base will protect the nail staining. Apply the base with as few strokes as possible – three strokes is the goal – the fewer the strokes the thinner the varnish.

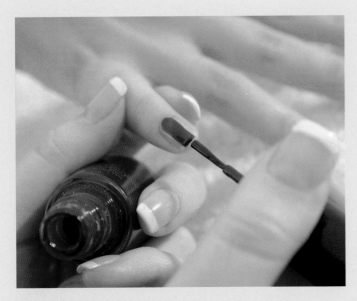

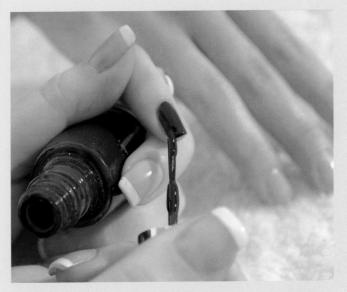

③ Before applying the colour make sure it is a good consistency. If a varnish is too thick dispose of it. Professional thinners can be bought and in an emergency a few drops of nail polish remover can be added to the bottle but it will change the pigment molecules in the varnish and thus weaken the finish.

④ Once the varnish is ready load the brush with varnish on one side only making sure the neck of the brush is clean of drips. Using three strokes of the brush, apply the colour down the centre and then on either side to completely cover the nail plate. Tidy any drips and splodges with a cotton bud tip soaked in varnish remover and move onto the second coat once the first coat on all nails is completed and dry.

⑤ Finally once you are happy with the colour application lock in and protect it with a top coat. The top coat will secure and maintain the colour for a lot longer than varnish alone as well as providing a shiny surface to finish. To fully complete the manicure wait until the varnish is nearly dry and apply a dry spray or layer of nail dryer to protect against smudges until the enamel is as hard as rock!

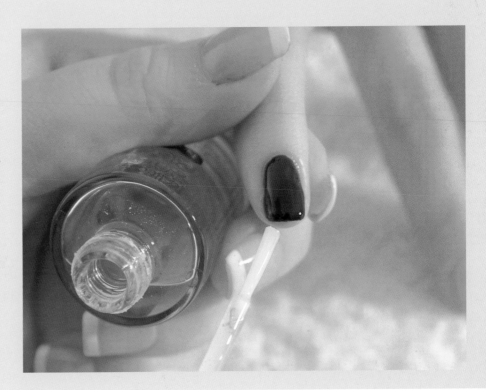

French manicure

The French manicure has been around for generations and is still immensely popular on natural and false nails. This natural, clean look shows nails in a healthy, glowing light and although the look seems tricky to achieve it can be very easy! All the rules of a normal manicure apply and need to be carried out before attempting the varnish application. French varnish can be troublesome when it comes to drying so the knack is to apply very thin layers.

The alternative to varnish is to use a white nail pencil to colour underneath the nails' free edge and create a great white look without the intricacies of a full French manicure.

This home manicure completed every seven to 10 days is great but if you want a special treat, then try a nail treatment like paraffin hot wax or a warm oil treatment at your local nail bar. Even hand masks and anti-ageing manicures are available so treat yourself occasionally and try one of the new up-and-coming treatments for hands and feet!

Professional therapy

Visiting a professional nail technician should be a pure delight, especially as there are so many treatments available nowadays to really pamper your hands. Warm waxes, oils and masks are utilised in many ways to really help improve the appearance of your hands and reverse the ageing process.

PARAFFIN WAX

Paraffin wax has been used for many years to warm and soothe the hands as well as locking in vital moisture during a manicure or pedicure. On the hands or feet this treatment is like no other. Warmed soft therapeutic wax is drizzled over the feet or hands and allowed to set like a mask for around 10 minutes. This warms the skin and soothes the muscles whilst boosting circulation to the bones and nerves. It is removed in a sheet and the warmed feet or hands are immediately massaged to encourage the absorption of the massage oil or lotion into the skin.

how to...

FRENCH MANICURE

This classic look suits all hands and leaves the nails looking clean and tidy. Practice makes perfect here, so don't give up. It's a difficult look to achieve but worth it when you do!

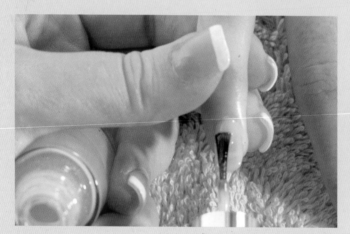

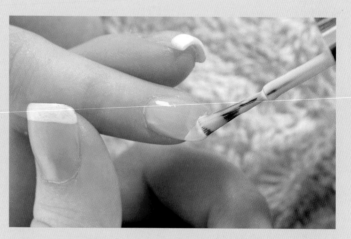

① Start by applying a good base coat (fingernails can go yellow even with a light pigmented varnish). For the best and most dramatic look, apply two coats of the pink base. French manicure pink can come in a variety of shades, from pinky beige to pinky red so choose the shade you prefer.

② Stroke on the white tips either with the help of pre-cut paper stencils or freehand. Using the stencils can ruin the pink base unless it is completely dry so try to master the freehand technique if you can. Seal and add gloss with a clear top coat.

PARAFFIN WAX

Warm wax is also great for relieving joint and muscular pain and proves to be generally therapeutic for hands and feet.

① **Place the hand over a plastic bag or a sheet of tin foil to protect your work surface.**

② **Ensure the wax is not too hot by testing it on the inside of your wrist first. When the temperature is just right, brush on or drizzle the warmed wax over the area, remembering to apply to the underside of the hand first. This is because the skin on the palm is thicker and needs a longer treatment time to achieve the same effect as on the back of the hand.**

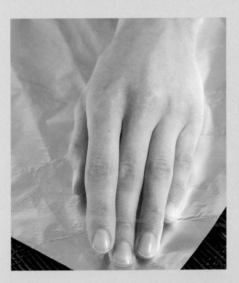
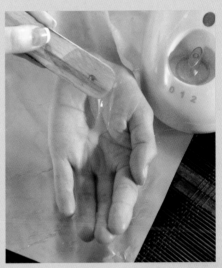

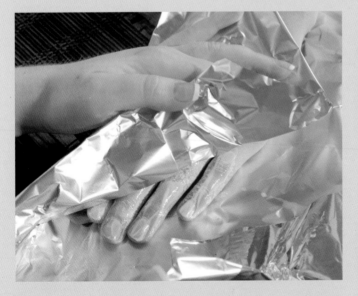
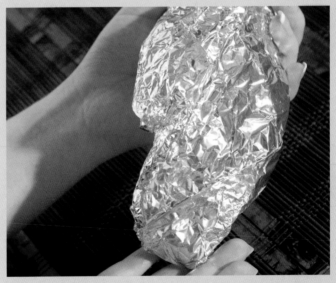

③ **Wrap the waxed area up in the foil or plastic bag and then a towel for about 10 minutes.**

④ **Unwrap the area and pull away the wax to reveal super soft, warm hands! Be aware of contra-indications as although the warm wax is good for dry skin, any open wounds will feel painful. Also, any contagious diseases could be encouraged to cross infect in the warm confined environment so avoid this treatment if you have any open wounds.**

WARM OIL CLOAK

This treatment is simple and very easy to carry out at home. Simply place a large bowl of very hot water on a flat surface and place a smaller bowl floating inside it. Pour a generous amount of sweet almond or macadamia nut oil inside the smaller bowl and wait for a few minutes until it warms. Place your fingers in the small bowl and allow them to soak for about five minutes. This really helps soften hardened cuticles and nails. After a few minutes rub the warm oil over the hands and up the arms to complete the massage routine. Oil will stay warm for a while so this added boost of nourishment will be really well absorbed by the skin. Hands can also be wrapped as with paraffin wax for 10 minutes if you have time for the extra moisturising factor! This warm oil treatment is equally luxurious on the feet and great for bad circulation.

MASKS AWAY!

The skin on the back of the hands is fine and is prone to sun damage, pigmentation changes and dryness, so applying a creamy, softening mask to the hands and leaving it to work for 10 minutes once a week can restore the moisture levels and help reinforce the skin's tone as well as boost its appearance dramatically.

Equally, a lightly scented tea tree or mint foot mask is great in the summer when cooled in the fridge. In the winter masks heated over a pan of warm water can snugly drench the toes with warmth and comfort – essential for those chilly nights! For an even bigger boost of warmth try thermal hand mitts. These are structured just like a thermal blanket and keep the hands snug for as long as you keep them on.

Anti-ageing treatments for nails can vary from masks and heat or spa treatments to serum applications. Most therapeutic treatments are very relaxing so why not try some new manicure treats and see what you think.

how to...

WARM OIL CLOAK

Taking the extra time to complete this treatment will reduce your cuticle work dramatically as they will be softened, thus making their removal easier.

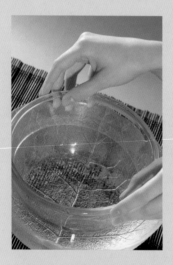 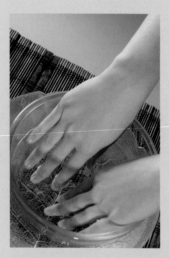 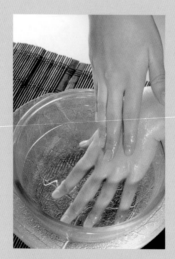 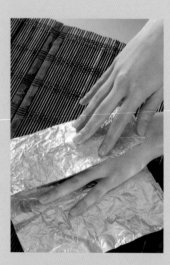

① Warm a small bowl of oil in a large bowl of hot water for a few minutes.

② Soak the dry skin area in the oil for five minutes.

③ Apply the warm oil over the hands and up the arms and follow the massage routine on pages 64–65.

④ Wrap the hands in foil to retain the heat and nourish the skin further.

The professional manicure

We often do our own nails and are happy to do so as we become more confident with what we like and practise how to achieve our favourite looks. A professional manicure will not be vastly different in principle to your own treatment as many of the steps you follow will also be adhered to by a nail technician. From New York to London, and Milan to Japan millions of people have their nails manicured every day and all for the same reasons: to relax, grab a coffee and enjoy the pamper!

It is in salons that you should expect to find hand and nail treatments such as paraffin wax and hot oil therapies but many offer spa treatments like LaStone® Therapy and deeper exfoliating treatments, too, so keep your eye out and try something new!

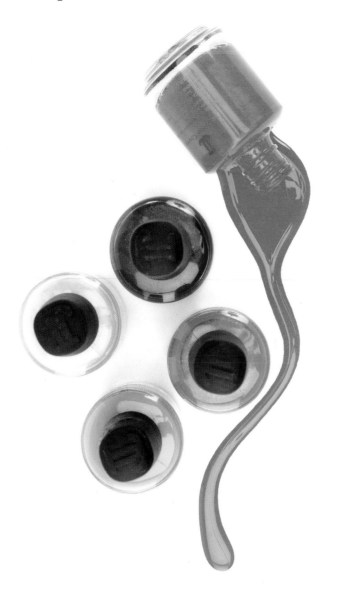

HERE IS WHAT YOU SHOULD AND SHOULDN'T EXPECT IN A NAIL SALON:

✓ Your nail technician should be clean and have freshly washed hands.

✓ The equipment being used on you must be sterilised before use.

✓ Your technician should tell you how much your treatment will cost and how long it will take.

✓ Your technician will analyse your nails and fill in a consultation card noting your nail type and which treatments are being carried out on that day.

✓ The salon should display a note of insurance to practice.

✓ Your technician should have qualifications in nail treatments or relevant experience.

✓ Your nail technician should be able to answer any technical questions you may have.

✗ Don't expect your treatment to finish on time. Remember your nails need to dry so allow time for this. When a quote on a nail treatment time is given it excludes dry time!

✗ Don't leave the salon having paid too much; the price quoted before the treatment or the one on the price list should not be added to regardless of the number of colours or glazes you have.

✗ Don't leave unsatisfied. Always say how you feel as your local salon would prefer you custom again.

✗ Don't have a treatment if you can see the tools and equipment are dirty as this can pass on infections from the previous client to you.

✗ Don't sit there in pain! Manicures should not painful. Even nail extensions should be comfortable to have put on so let the technician know if a treatment is painful or too hot.

The male manicure

A manicure performed on a man is similar to one performed on a woman but for a few minor differences. There is usually no nail varnish required and top nail primer is used instead of base coat as it is a matt and invisible strengthener that treats the nails. Nail masks are also used to treat the nails individually as often men use their hands more roughly than women. The nail filing will be natural and follow the shape of the fingertip and the hands must be well moisturised with a water-based cream to leave the skin nourished but non-greasy. More emphasis is on buffing with men as they will see the finished result as opposed to women who will likely wear varnish or at least a top coat to protect their nails. The majority of my clients in London are men having grooming treatments and there are now many spas and salons dedicated to men-only therapy. Most of my clients are in the public eye and on television and so it is vital to appear well-groomed. The following manicure will leave any hands feeling soft and supple.

NAIL MASKS...

All professional nail treatments are used on men, too, so experimenting with different massage treatments or masks will be fun and can only improve the appearance of nails and hands. Nail masks are great for restoring moisture to the nail plate without the need for a time-consuming treatment which you may not have time for. Simply paint on the mask and wear it for a few hours until it is time to peel it off. Usually active ingredients such as orange and avocado are found in these products and they really give the nails a soft texture.

how to...

MALE MANICURE

Turn into modern man and get grooming with this simple manicure treatment!

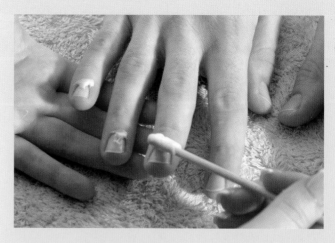

① **Wash your hands and pat dry to remove daily build-up of dirt and perspiration. Apply small blobs of cuticle cream to the cuticles and massage in to warm the skin around the base of the nails and to allow it to sink into the cuticles.**

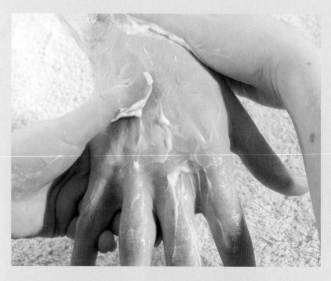

② **Follow the guidelines for the massage on pages 64–65 and apply as much pressure as you feel is needed to release the tension in the muscles and to soothe the joints. If you have calluses, then the massage can be focused around them for their later removal.**

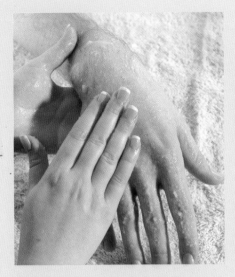

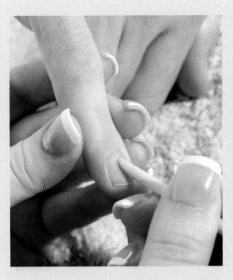

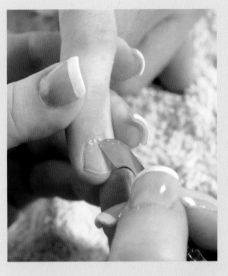

③ Exfoliate the hands without washing off the cream and soak the nails. Rinse then dry. If you suffer from calluses, either use a pumice to smooth the surface of the skin or a chemical-based hard skin remover to soften the skin and turn it white so you can buff off the dry skin. Massage a little cream in to finish.

④ Push back cuticles with an orange wood stick or hoof stick and clip away any excess cuticle skin with the nippers.

⑤ Using the cuticle knife, gently work with circular movements to lift and release the cuticles from the nail plate. The skin should now be very soft so this process should be easy.

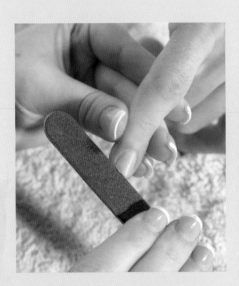

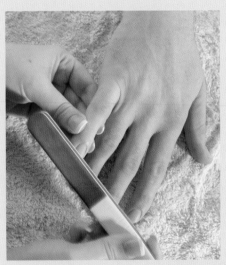

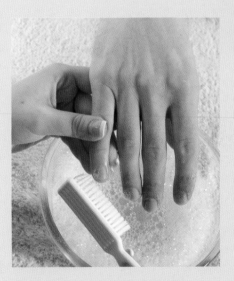

⑥ File the nails into a shape that mirrors the natural shape of the end of the fingers or the lunula. Bevel with the file to remove fuzzy nail edges and buff to finish the filing process.

⑦ Using the block buffer or multi-side buffer, work to bring about a super shine with the roughest side first and the smoothest last.

⑧ Brush the nails and remove any excess dirt from under the fingernails with an orange stick or cotton bud. Apply a matt nail treatment to suit the nail type and help maintain it strength.

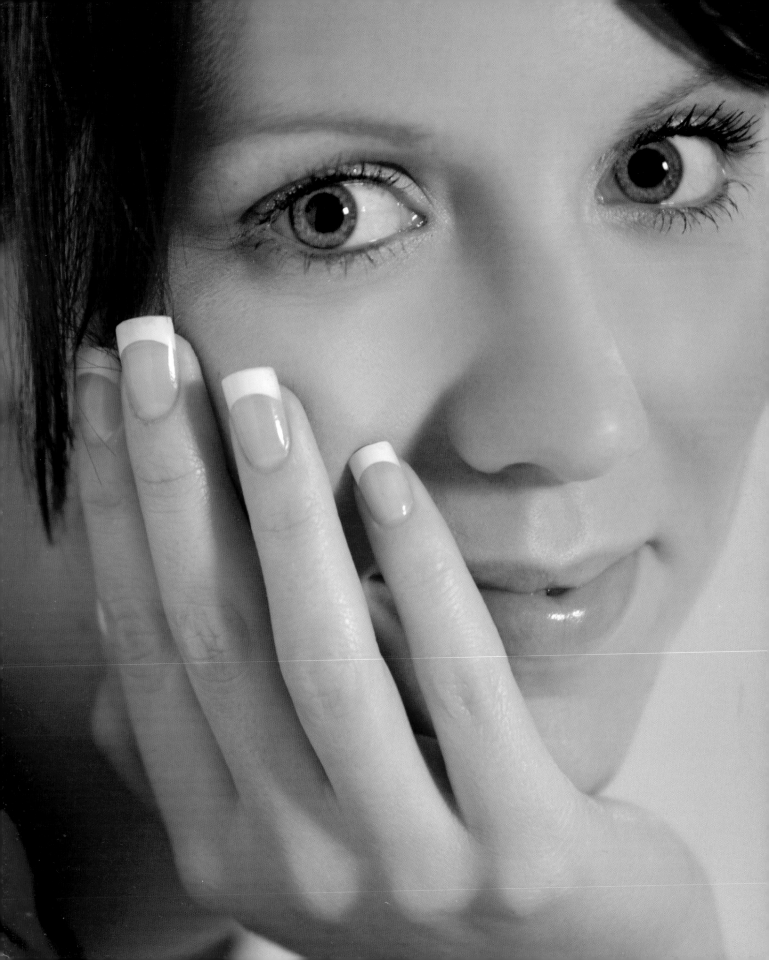

07 artificial nails

artificial nails

Strong, healthy natural nails are great if you have them but what if you don't? Artificial nails add length to your nails but still look natural. The best of both worlds and as strong a steel, these nails really do all the hard work for you.

Artificial nails have been worn for thousands of years. Even in Egyptian times gold nails were stuck onto natural nails as a sign of wealth. It was America, however, that first made artificial nails big business and today millions of Americans regularly have nail extensions, many of which have not seen their natural nails for years!

Three main systems are used to create the hard outer surface to artificial nails. It is this surface which gives the nails their lasting strength. Each of these systems has both advantages and disadvantages and it is up to the client to decide which works best for them. The systems are those of acrylic, fibreglass or silk and gel. Each is very strong and durable but for one reason or another you will probably have a preference.

Acrylic

Acrylic is the most popular bonding used as an over-layer to strengthen nail extensions and it currently captures over 70 per cent of the nail market. Acrylic was first used by dentists to mould dentures but was found to give great strength to nails, too! Pink and white colourings are added to the acrylic to create different looks but the majority of clients opt of a clear, translucent finish.

The acrylic system is a combination of two substances: a powder containing benzoyl peroxide and a liquid containing amine (a chemical compound). When they are mixed together they act as a catalyst for the monomers in both products to react and create a gel substance that hardens to the surface we see on the nails in a matter of seconds. EMA (ethyl methacrylate) is a popular monomer and is present in most nail products.

When the acrylic mixture dries it is extremely strong and nail technicians apply the mixture in layers to add extra strength. Once plastic nail tips have been applied for added length the acrylic mixture of powder and liquid is applied to coat and form the nail itself.

Acrylic is a great system because it is quick, strong and looks natural if applied properly. The downsides are that it is smelly, messy and the acrylic is often so hard that any bangs to the nails can result in tremendous pain! These are long-lasting nails and need infilling every two to three weeks. Removing them requires melting the acrylic with acetone which takes a while and is expensive. They last for between three and six weeks.

There are three ways of applying acrylic to the nail: on top of a nail extension; applied to your natural nail to add strength; or applied to the free edge of your nail to add length and then over the whole nail for strength.

In theory, the application of acrylic nails is relatively simple, in practice, however, it is very difficult to do well!

trade secrets

- Always keep your tools clean and dust-free. A nail technician's nail brush should be cleaned for every client and left to dry naturally to prevent it going hard.

- Wear a face mask if possible as the fumes can trigger a migraine after hours of use. Long-term, it can also affect your sense of smell, so protect yourself.

- Spend time practising creating an acrylic ball; it is important to get the perfect mix of powder and liquid.

- Speed is of the essence, so concentrate when applying the acrylic; the smallest slip and you will spend hours filing away mistakes.

- Practise applying thin layers, as one thick layer will not be strong enough and can be brittle.

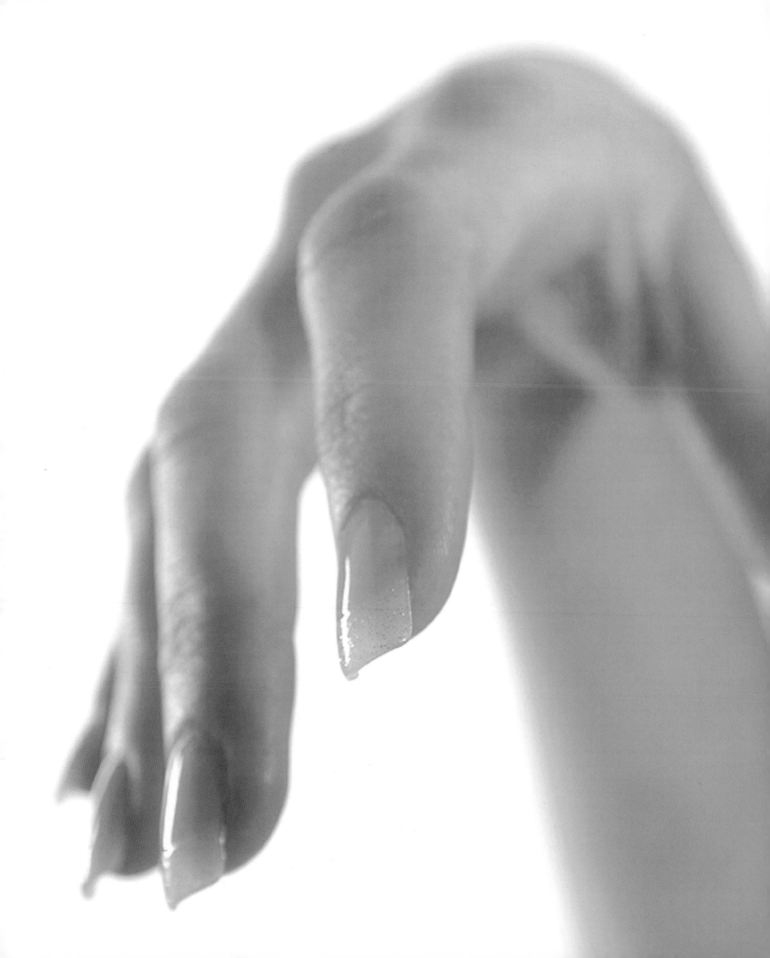

THE TOOLS FOR ACRYLICS

① 100/180 grit buffer
② Cuticle oil
③ Extension clippers
④ Cotton wool discs
⑤ Block buffer
⑥ Nail form
⑦ Acrylic brush
⑧ Cuticle stick
⑨ Acrylic powders

▽ *Some nail tools can be expensive but bear in mind they will last for a long time if looked after properly so they will be a good investment. Quality overrides quality when it comes to tools!*

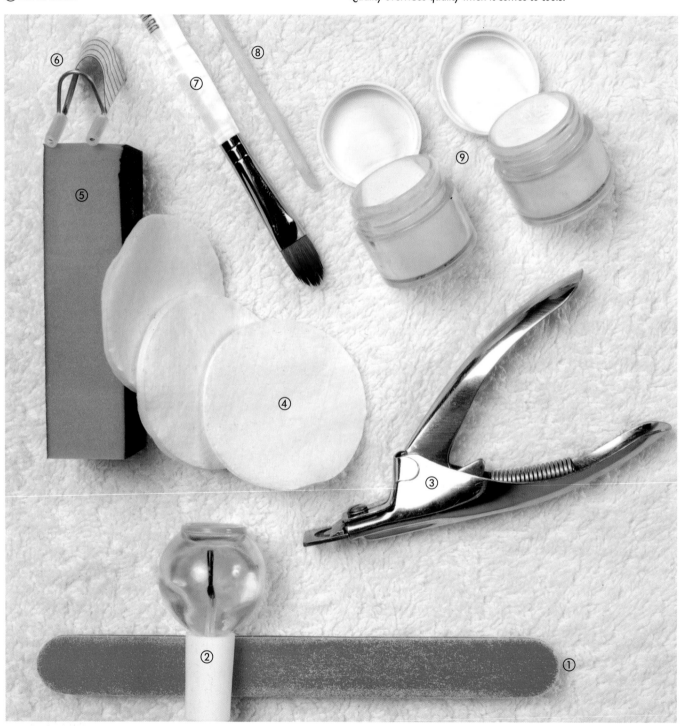

how to...

AMAZING ACRYLIC

Acrylic nails have been worn by millions of women for many years and are still the most requested type of nail extension because they are amazingly durable and look quite natural.

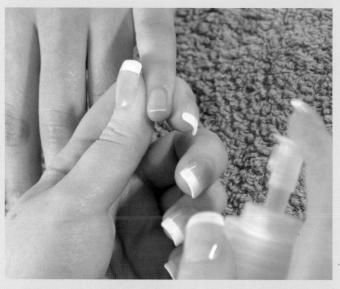

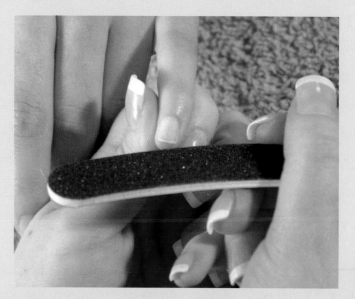

① Clean the nails of varnish and sanitise them thoroughly to ensure there is no bacteria lying on the surface of the nails. If the cuticles are long it is an idea to push them back now to prevent damage when filing which can catch the skin and tear the cuticles.

② File the natural nails down to prolong the life of the extensions. Bevel to remove any fluffy edges after filing or block buff. Scuff the whole surface of the nails with the finer side of a nail file. The nail plate is very thin so if it feels hot, then you have filed too much away!

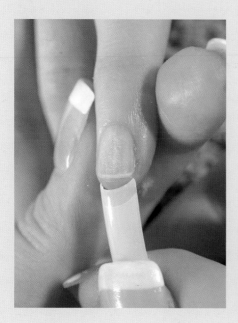

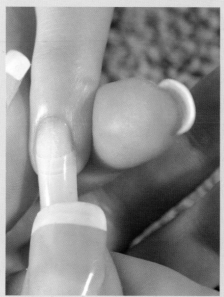

③ Once all the nail plates are rough and dull, size your extension tips to the width and curvature of the natural nail, ensuring they are an exact match by filing any excess tip away where it is not needed. Apply the tip after filling the lower edge of the nail with adhesive nail glue. With very light pressure and ensuring no air bubbles have formed under the surface of the tip (as these can lead to infection), place and push the tip onto the nail just below the free edge. Alternatively, place the tip half way down the nail and stick it in place. This will make a stronger nail but will create a less natural end result.

artificial nails **83**

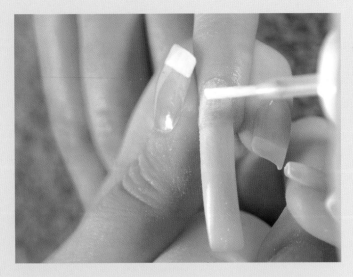

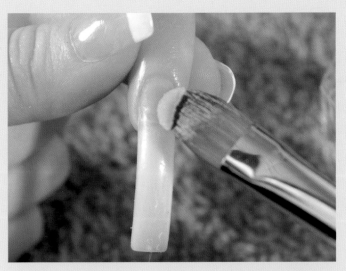

④ File across the base of the plastic extension until there is no noticeable line between the extension and the natural nail. To ensure a sterile environment spray the nails regularly with antibacterial spray to neutralise bacteria. The spray will evaporate quickly leaving you with a clean working surface. Remove the excess nail dust from the nail by firstly brushing with a large nail brush and then wipe the plates with varnish remover to ensure they are clean of debris which could affect the acrylic application. Dot some nail primer onto the nails. This is an irritant substance which aids the attachment of acrylic to the nail. Be sure not to get it on to the skin as it will sting although no damage will be done.

⑤ Hold the nail firmly and dip the brush into the acrylic liquid. Once the brush is saturated remove the excess by pressing it to the side of the glass dish and dip the tip of the brush into the acrylic powder. Once the powder is wet you have a matter of 20 seconds to mould the acrylic before it starts to harden, so work quickly.

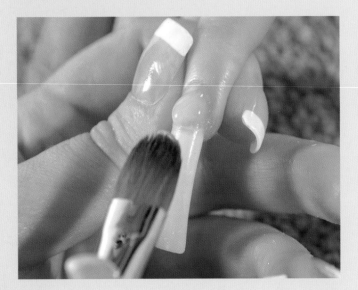

⑥ Apply a small ball to the tip of the nail where the tip join is. Place a second ball close to the cuticle and smooth over the whole nail. Repeat this move with a third ball and finish with a ball on the tip again but brush backwards from tip to cuticle when the ball is on the tip.

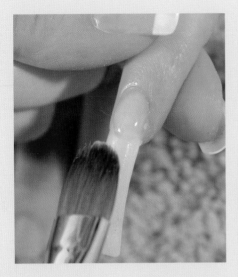

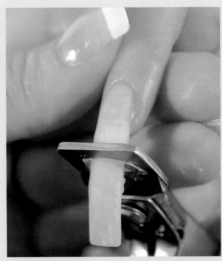

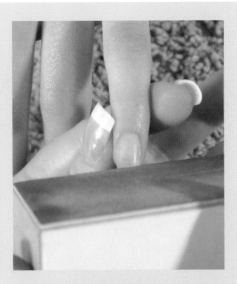

⑦ The acrylic can be manipulated but allowing it to run a little down the nail can help you apply a smooth coat. Allow the acrylic to dry for 30 seconds. When dry, the nail will feel very hard. Using the 100/180 grit boomerang, buff the roughness of the nail all over and file the free edge again if necessary.

⑧ Using the nail extension clippers, cut the length you do not require off the extension and shape the end to suit your style: either square, sqoval, round or oval. Artificial nails are stronger than natural nails and you don't need to consider weak points so pick your preferred nail shape as they will all be strong!

⑨ After the nail plate has been smoothed and there are no visible gaps or joins, work the block buffer over the nails, refining the surface of the acrylic until it is completely smooth.

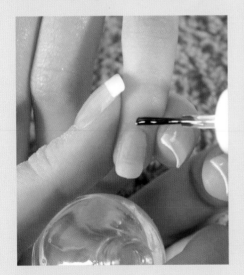

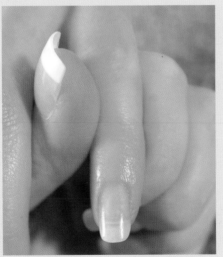

AND LASTLY...

Acrylic does look very natural but because it is slightly opaque you can tell the nails are artificial close-up so I would always recommend a varnish, even if it is just an almost clear French manicure pink.

⑩ Apply a little cuticle oil to the skin on the fingers to ensure they are well nourished and allow to absorb for a few minutes before washing the hands thoroughly.

⑪ Once the hands are clean and dry apply the varnish of your choice and top coat to seal the colour.

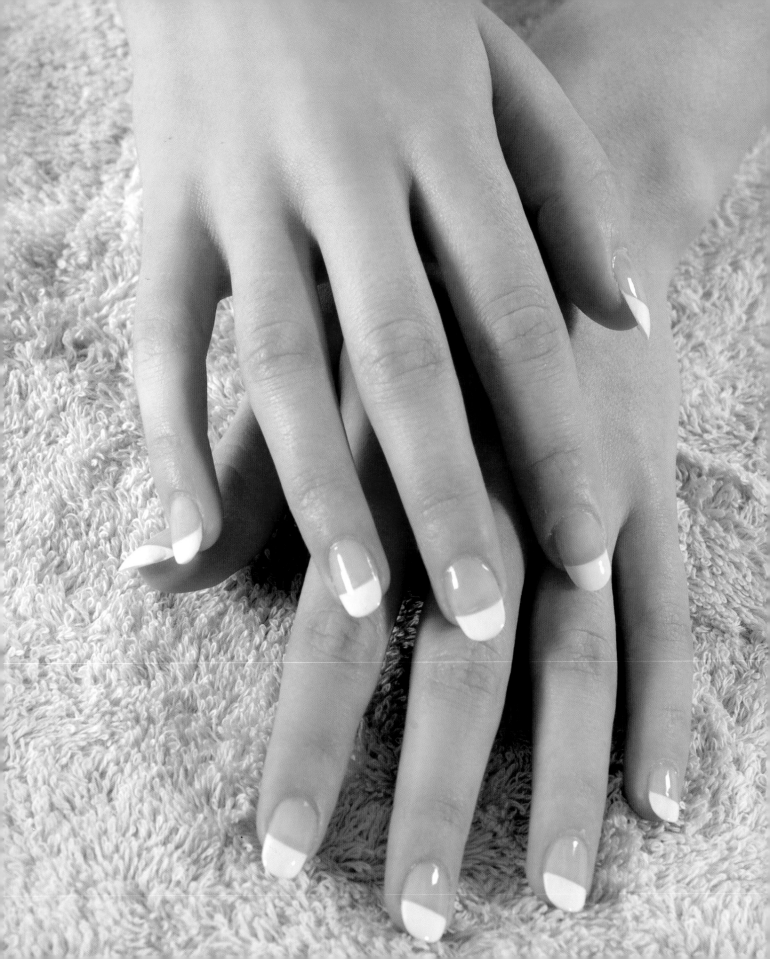

how to...

ACRYLIC FORMING

Acrylic can be used as an overlay on top of, or building onto, natural nails. This follows the exact same process as applying a plastic tip but instead a foil form is used to shape the wet acrylic to give it the shape your nail would naturally grow. This method works well on nails that already have a little free edge. The end result is very natural and often wearers don't apply a varnish, instead they favour just a buffed shiny finish and some cuticle oil to nourish the surrounding skin post treatment.

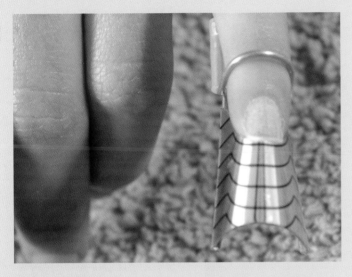

① **Prepare the nails as in Steps 1 and 2 (see page 83). Attach the nail form so that the foil rests under the free edge.**

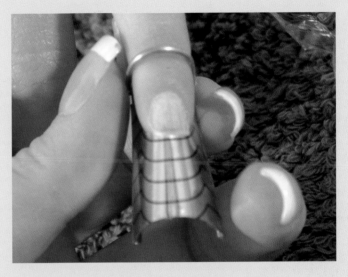

② **Scuff the nail and apply primer. Prepare to apply the acrylic to the free edge.**

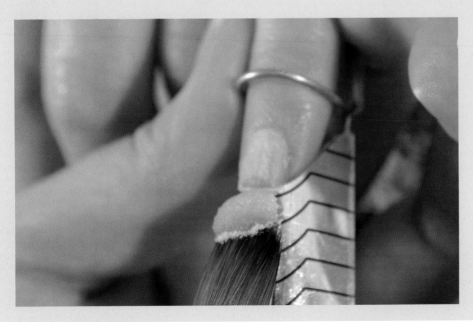

③ **Ball the acrylic and powder and place it on the free edge. Build up the acrylic layers over the entire nail plate and manipulate to create a new nail.**

Gel

The gel system produces the most natural looking finish as the gel is completely transparent. It is known as a pre-mixed system because unlike acrylic no mixing is necessary. The gel is just one substance which is set with UV light.

Nail gels do not harden in the presence of oxygen and so the extra UV light is required to act as the catalyst to allow the gel to harden. Most gels leave a slightly sticky surface after drying but if this is wiped away correctly it is not a problem. Some gels have a very thin consistency and these are best used as top layers due to their shiny appearance or to build up thin layers on natural nails for extra strength. Thicker gels carry more strength and are better for use with extensions.

The preparation for gel nails is virtually the same as acrylic but the overall effect is more natural but less hardwearing.

THE TOOLS FOR GEL

① 100/180 grit boomerang file
② Cuticle oil
③ Block buffer
④ Gel brush
⑤ Crystal nail file
⑥ Cotton wool discs
⑦ Extension clippers
⑧ Gel

▽ *Gel nails are delicate and look the most realistic of the three types. The equipment is specially designed for the gel substance and all these tools must be bought to complete the treatment.*

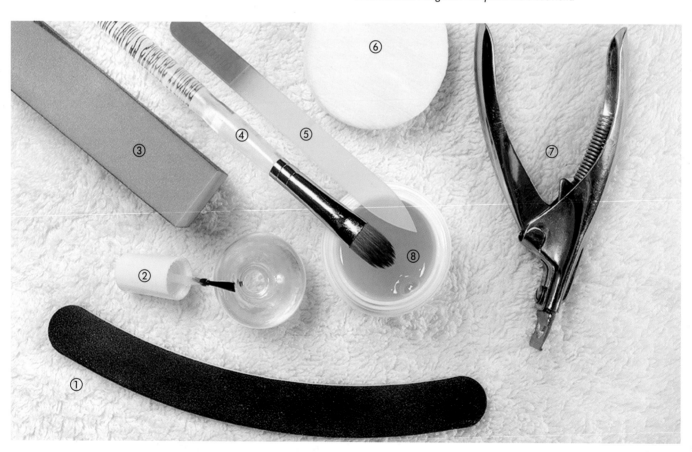

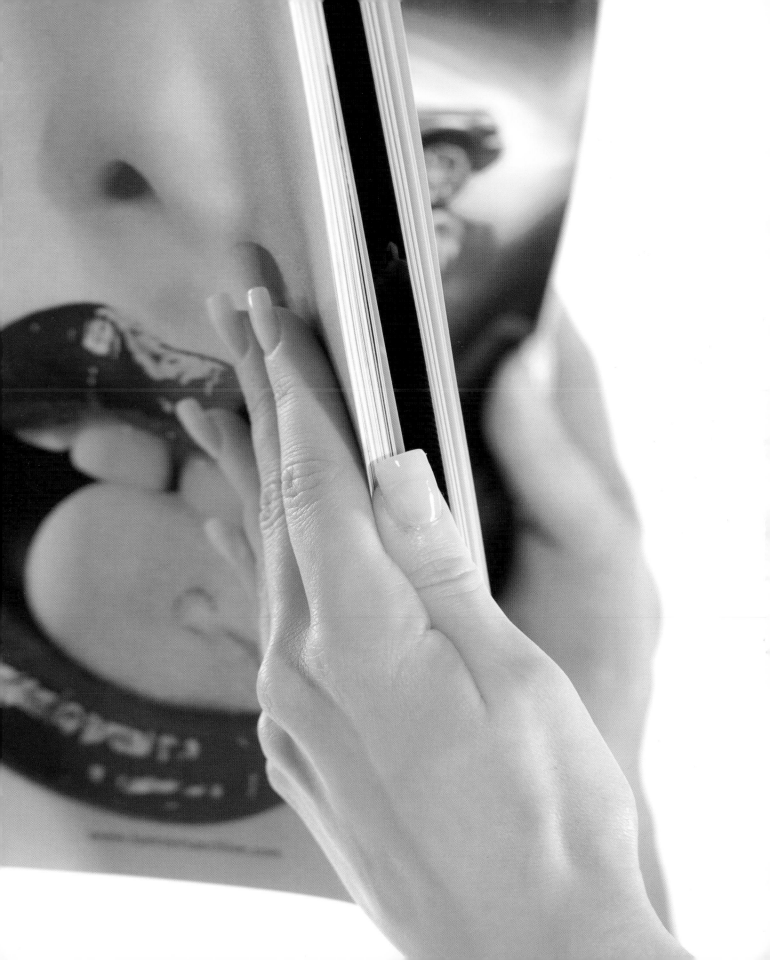

how to...

GORGEOUS GEL

It is hard to identify gel nails when they are applied well and although not known for being the strongest of the three methods, gel is a popular choice for many women because of its natural look.

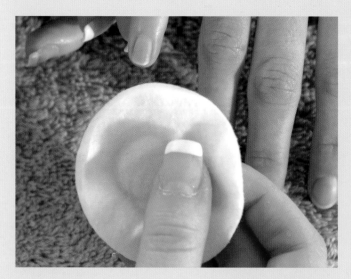

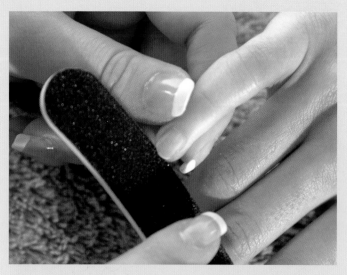

① Clean the nails of varnish and sanitise them thoroughly to ensure there is no bacteria lying on the surface of the nail. If the cuticles are long, push them back now.

② File the natural nails down to prolong the life of the extensions. Bevel to remove any fluffy edges after filing or block buff.

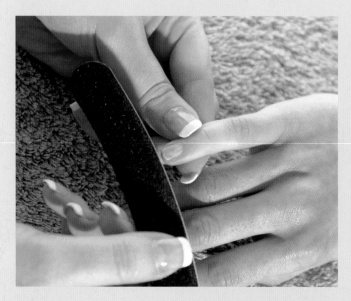

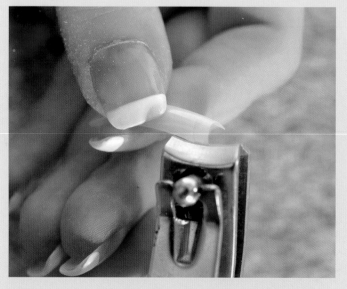

③ Scuff the whole surface of the nails with the finer side of the nail file. The nail plate is very thin so stop filing if it starts to feel hot.

④ Once all the nail plates are rough and dull, size your extension tips to the width of the nails, ensuring they are an exact match by filing or clipping away any excess tip.

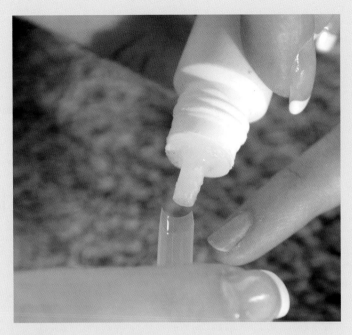

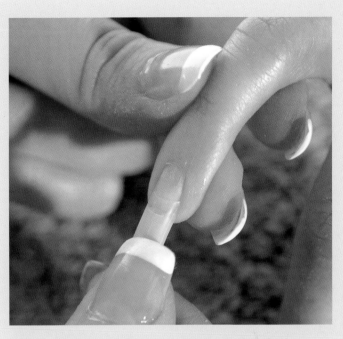

⑤ Apply the tip after filling the lower edge of the extension with adhesive nail glue.

⑥ With very light pressure and ensuring no air bubbles have formed under the surface of the tip (as these can lead to infection), place the tip and push it onto nail just below the free edge.

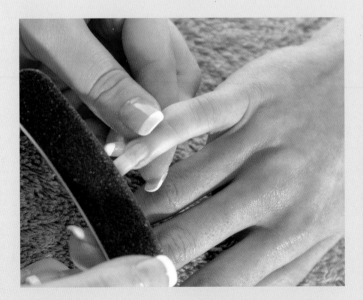

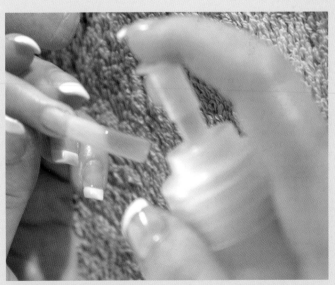

⑦ File across the base of the plastic extension until there is no noticeable line between the extension and the natural nail.

⑧ Spray the nails regularly with antibacterial spray to neutralise bacteria. The spray will evaporate quickly leaving you with a clean working surface.

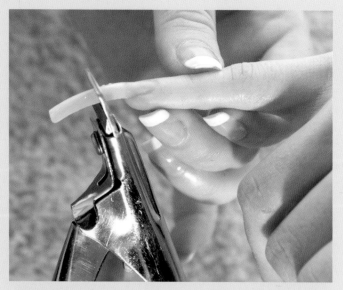

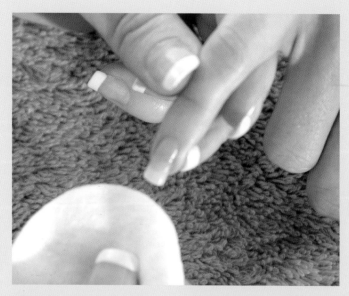

⑨ Cut the length you do not require off the extension and shape the end of the shortened nail to suit your needs: either square, sqoval, round or oval. Remember that artificial nails are much stronger than natural nails and you don't need to consider weak points so freely pick your preferred nail shape as they will all be strong!

⑩ Remove the excess nail dust by brushing with a large nail brush and then wipe the plates with varnish remover to ensure they are clean of debris which could affect the gel application.

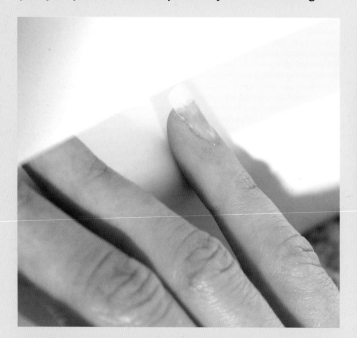

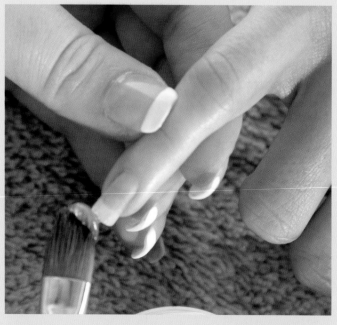

⑪ Switch on the UV light and start applying the gel to four fingers of one hand only. A thin coat will do as a base, just be sure not to get any gel on the skin. Place the four gelled fingertips under the light for two minutes, after which repeat the procedure on the other hand.

⑫ Repeat the application three times so each nail has three layers of gel, including the thumbs. There may be a sticky residue on the nails after the final curing under the lamp. Gently wipe this away with a nail cloth.

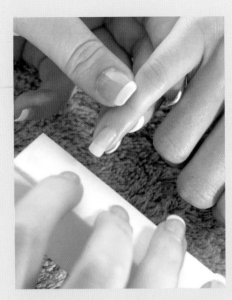

⑬ Using a nail file or just the buffer, smooth the surface of the nail until it is even and buff to a high shine.

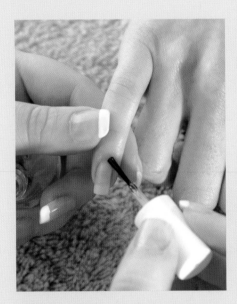

⑭ Apply cuticle oil to the skin to re-nourish and wash the hands to clean away all debris. Leave the nails as they are and apply a top coat or varnish with your choice of colour to finish. Finally apply a top coat over the varnish to increase the durability of the colour.

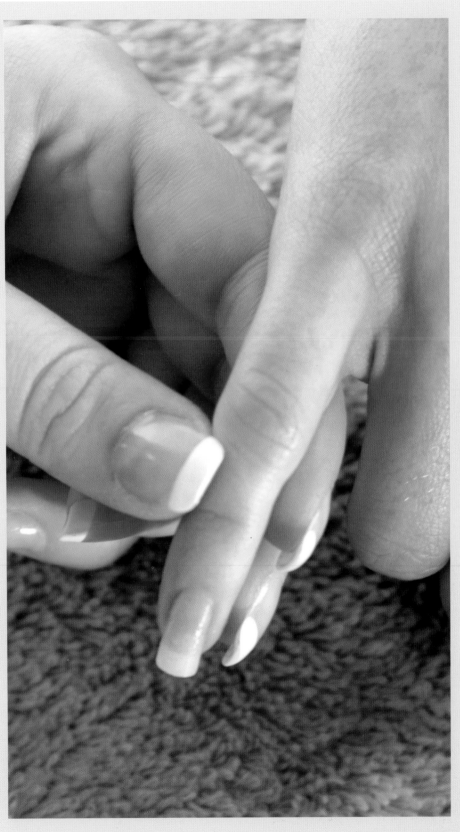

Fibreglass and silk

Developed by beauty therapists, the fibreglass system was born after a stronger alternative to glue and tissue paper was needed for mending nail breaks and splits. The three-component system of fibreglass or silk mesh, resin and resin activator allows the nail technician to build up natural nails and layer on layer provide a strong and sturdy extension.

Personal preference will indicate whether you use silk or fibreglass and both are very strong. The silk mesh is sticky on one side so it can be easily applied to the nail in a strip from cuticle to tip. Fibreglass is slightly more durable but does not disappear when dampened by the resin whereas silk almost totally disappears and becomes one with the resin so can look more natural. The resin used is a chemical of the acrylic family but it will dry and harden when exposed to air alone. Ethyl cyanoacrylate is a popular choice for resin and it is used in many industries as a reliable adhesive for wood, metal and piping!

Activator spray is used to speed up the process of hardening the resin as naturally it takes about 15 minutes. The activator cuts this time down to a few seconds but if applied incorrectly it can be very uncomfortable and burn the skin. The spray must be applied from a 30 cm (12 in) distance as if sprayed too close the skin can feel like it is burning or irritated. Along with this uncomfortable reaction the resin will crack and produce a weak overlay with many tiny cracks.

THE TOOLS FOR FIBREGLASS AND SILK

① **Fibreglass/silk sheets**
② **Block buffer**
③ **Cotton wool discs**
④ **Cuticle oil**
⑤ **3-way final polish buffer**
⑥ **Extension clippers**

▷ *Silk and fibreglass require quality rather than quantity when it comes to tools. Pre-cut fibres and silk now make the job of sizing the fibre much easier, so use them!*

trade secrets

- Do not breathe in or get resin or activator in your eye as it will sting and medical attention will be needed immediately. If you wish, try wearing a nose and mouth mask to prevent breathing in too many particles.

- To ensure the mesh cannot be seen through the resin make sure you wet the mesh thoroughly on the first application otherwise the end result will be unnatural and the mesh very visible.

- When applying the mesh leave a little gap around the edge of the whole nail as this will provide a much more natural look to the nail when finished.

- Do not over buff as the resin may be filed away quickly and expose the precious mesh which will look terrible and often the nail will have to be done again.

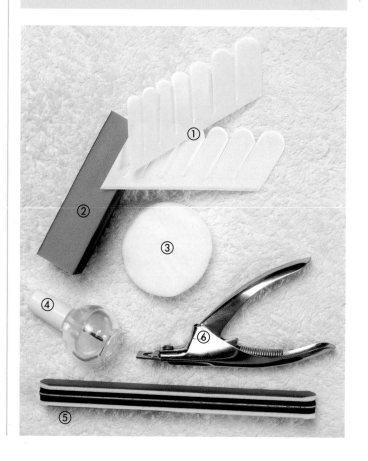

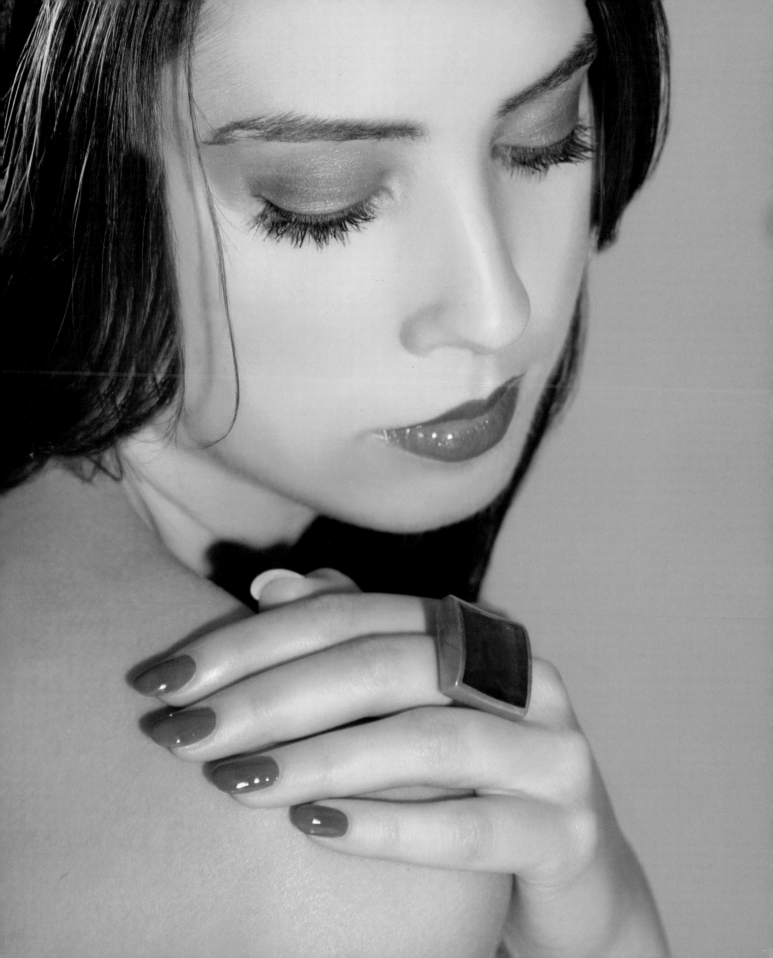

how to...

FIBREGLASS OR SILK

Not only superb for mending breaks but over extensions, fibreglass/silk provides a strong, natural finish to the nails.

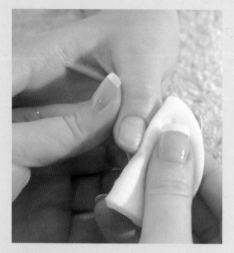

① Clean the nails of varnish and sanitise them thoroughly to ensure there is no bacteria lying on the surface of the nails. If the cuticles are long push them back now.

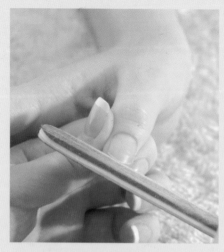

② File the natural nails down to prolong the life of the extensions. Bevel to remove any fluffy edges after filing or block buff.

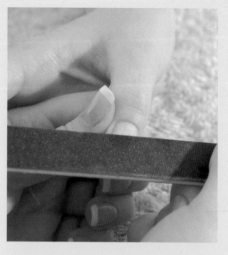

③ Scuff the whole surface of the nails with the finer side of the nail file. The nail plate is very thin so if it feels hot, then you have filed too much away.

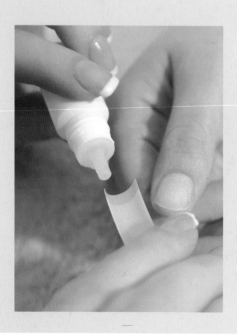

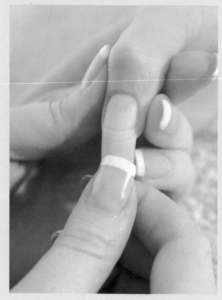

④ Once all the nail plates are rough and dull, size your extension tips to the width of the nails, ensuring they are an exact match by filing any excess tip away. Apply the tip after filling the lower edge of the artificial nail with adhesive nail glue. With very light pressure and ensuring no air bubbles have formed under the surface of the tip (as these can lead to infection) place and push the tip onto the nail just below the free edge. Alternatively place the tip half way down the nail and stick it in place. This will make a stronger nail but will create a less natural end result.

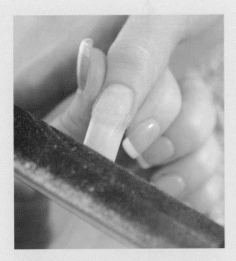

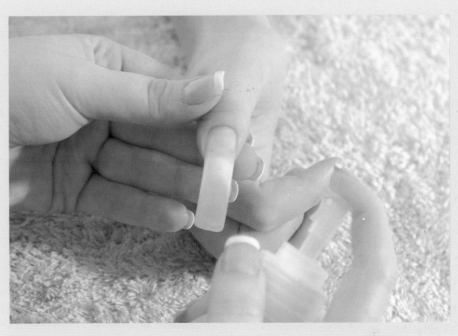

⑤ File across the base of the plastic extension until there is no noticeable line between the extension and the natural nail.

⑥ To ensure a sterile environment spray the nails regularly with antibacterial spray which will neutralise bacteria. The spray will evaporate quickly leaving you with a clean working surface.

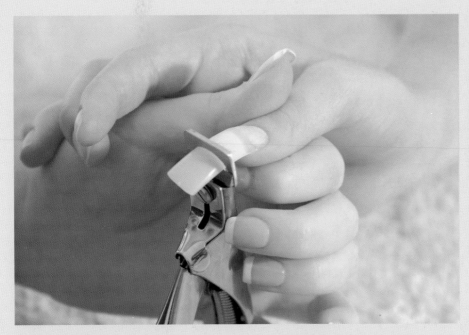

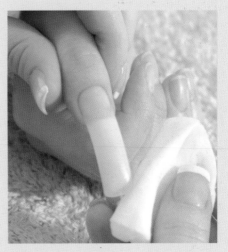

⑦ Cut the length you do not require off the extension and shape the end of the shortened nail to suit your needs: either square, sqoval, round or oval. Remember that artificial nails are much stronger than natural nails and you don't need to consider weak points so freely pick your preferred nail shape as they will all be strong!

⑧ Remove the excess nail dust from the nail by brushing with a large nail brush and then wipe the plates with varnish remover to ensure they are clean of debris which could affect the fibreglass or silk application.

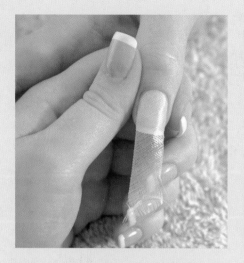
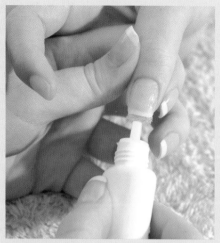
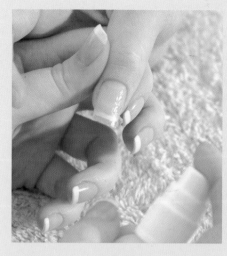

⑨ Apply the mesh to the nail with the sticky side on the nail plate, leaving a small gap around the sides and cuticle of the nail. Pre-cut fibres are now available which speeds up the process as no cutting and shaping is necessary.

⑩ Cut the excess fibre away and wet with the first layer of resin. Spray at 30 cm (12 in) to activate the resin when you are sure it is all wet and has turned transparent. Make sure there is no resin on the skin before spraying as this will cause irritation. Apply the second coat of resin and spray followed by a third and final coat of resin and spray to activate the hardening process. If the nozzle clogs, replace it or try a brush on product it you find them easier.

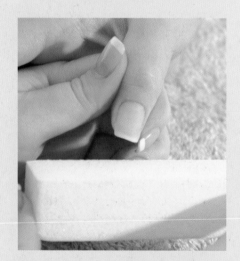
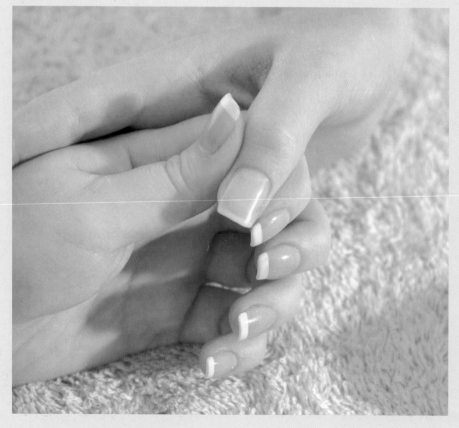

⑪ Once the three coats are dry file lightly to remove unevenness with the nail file, then block buff with the buffer to smooth and complete the treatment. Varnish to finish or buff to a shine if you prefer the natural look.

how to...

MENDING BREAKS

Splits, cracks and breaks on natural nails can all be mended and treated by using either acrylic, gel or fibreglass nail systems. Often the better choice is fibreglass as this is what it was originally invented for and works well in localised areas.

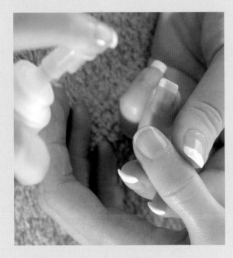

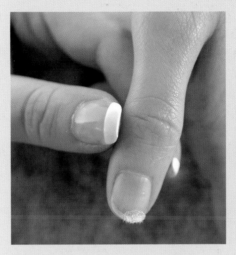

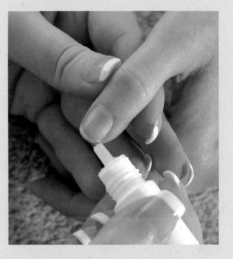

① Clean the nails of debris or old nail varnish using some varnish remover and sanitising spray. Cotton wool can stick in the nail break so a tissue works well here.

② Start by glueing the split together then cut a small piece of fibreglass or silk and apply it to the break ensuring it completely covers both sides of the tear.

③ Just like the fibreglass method of applying extensions, apply the resin and activator spray in two layers on the small piece of fibreglass used to cover the break.

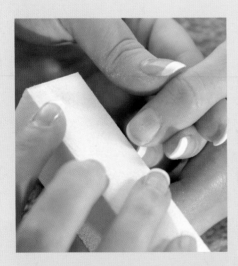

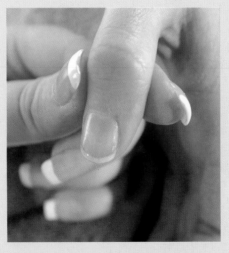

④ Once the resin is dry from the second layer, lightly buff to ensure it is as smooth as the natural nail and there is no obvious rough edge to the mended tear.

⑤ Varnish as usual to complete the tear and get the nail properly fixed with an extension or acrylic overlay as soon as possible to prevent further tearing.

AND LASTLY...

Dipping fingers in acetone will remove acrylic and fibreglass nails by breaking down the bond of chemicals that make them and melting them off. However, gel nails are not easily removed by soaking and will require buffing off. Go gently and have regular breaks to allow the nails to cool.

Never pick or leaver off nail extensions or overlays. Always soak in acetone to avoid damage to the natural nails.

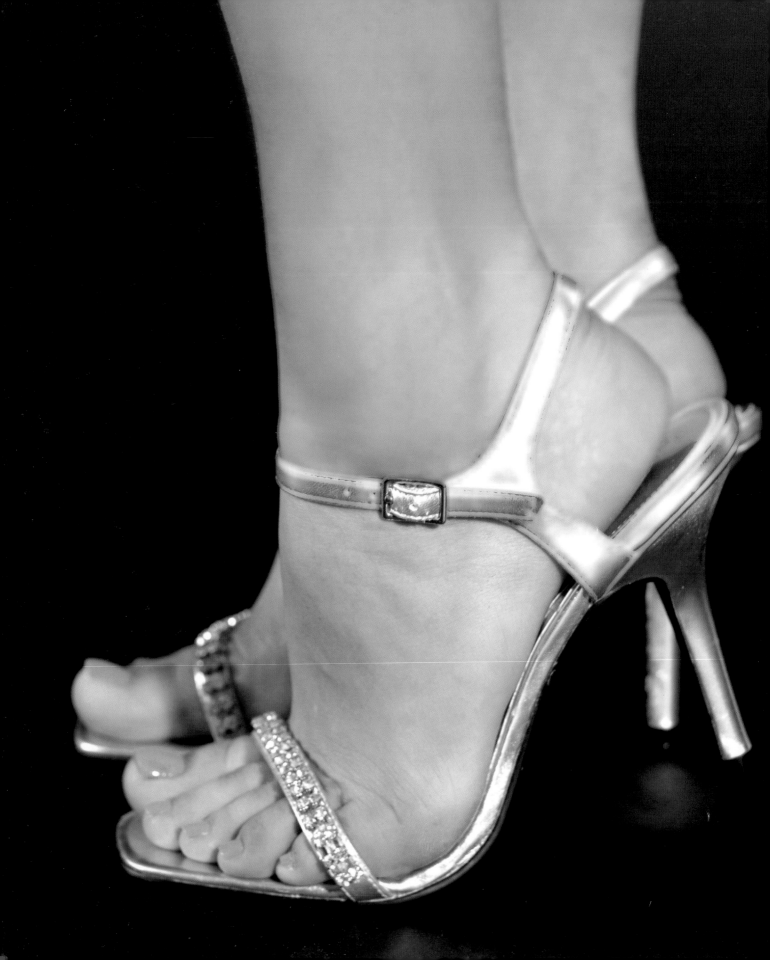

the pedicure

The Pedicure

Pedicures are just as popular as manicures and are no longer only reserved for the summer months. Smooth, well-groomed feet are very attractive and with the fashions in footwear becoming increasingly bare we find ourselves exposing our feet more than ever.

Both men and women are taking steps to improve the appearance of their feet. A professional pedicure involves far more than simply cutting toenails. A de-stress massage and vital exfoliation are performed to prevent ankles swelling and to improve the look and feel of unsightly rough skin. Looking after feet is very important as they carry the weight of the body every day for many hours.

A pedicure treatment in a nail bar will take approximately 45 minutes with additional drying time. A home pedicure should take around 30 minutes and should be performed every two weeks.

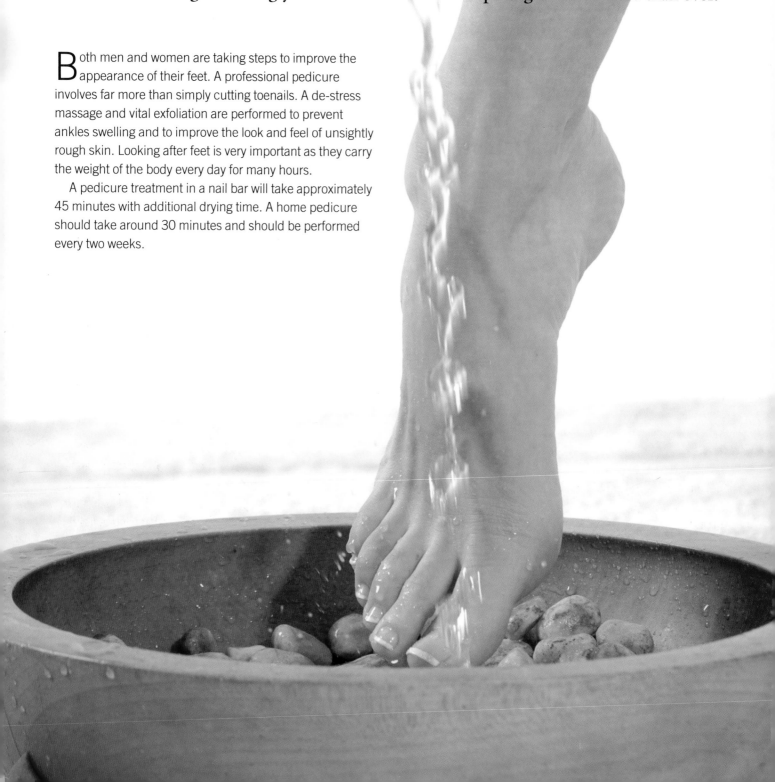

how to...

THE HOME PEDICURE

Performing a self-pedicure not only improves the appearance of feet but is very relaxing and give you vital pamper time!

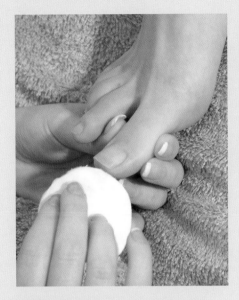

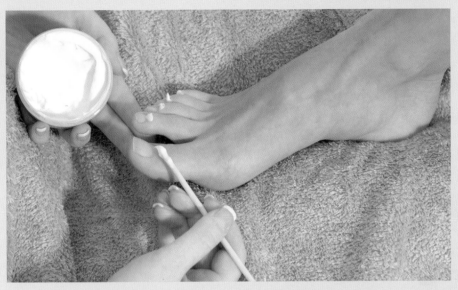

① Start by sterilising your tools and placing them on tissue paper. Wash your hands and relax in a chair that allows you to comfortably reach your feet. If your toes are varnished, dampen a cotton pad with non-acetone nail varnish remover and hold over the nails for 10 seconds before wiping off the free edge to cleanly remove all excess varnish on the nail plate. Use a cotton bud dipped in varnish remover to get into the nail wall and under the free edge if necessary.

② Apply a pea size amount of cuticle cream to the cuticles and rub in before soaking the feet in a bowl or spa of warm water. Because the skin on the soles of the feet is particularly rough, the longer the feet soak in water the softer the hard skin becomes and therefore easier to remove. For added benefit, add a tablespoonful coarse sea salt, a teaspoon of milk and three drops of essential oil of peppermint, eucalyptus or geranium to the warm foot spa to create a fresh and balancing environment.

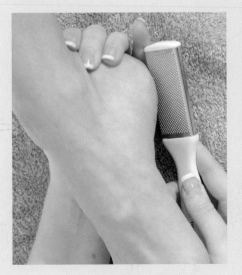

③ Remove the feet from the spa and pat dry. Using a metal foot rasp, gently remove the hard skin from areas on the heels, toes and balls of the feet. Do not rub too vigorously as this will remove too much skin and possibly cause breaks in the skin which will leave it open to infection. Instead keep checking the area until you can no longer feel the build up of hard skin. The rasp will remove the hard skin but will also leave it feeling rough so buff to a smooth finish. Use the fine foot buff or pumice to remove any excess rough surfaces.

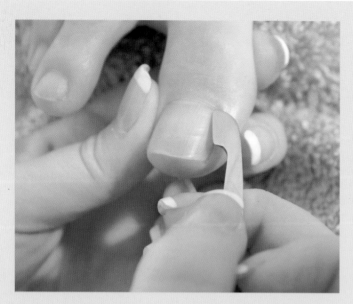

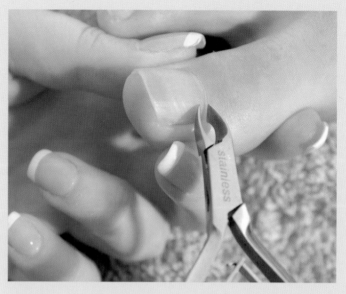

④ Use a cuticle knife or orange wood stick to push back the cuticles and remove any surface cuticle cells from the nail plate.

⑤ Excess cuticle may need to be trimmed off with cuticle nippers but be sure to leave a little amount to protect the matrix from damage. Removing too much cuticle may contribute to nail damage.

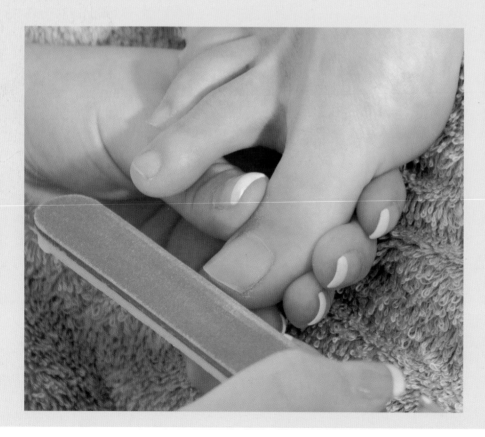

⑥ Next, trim the free edge and file the nails into shape. The best shape for toenails is square as they look fantastic and also help to keep the nails from in-growing which can be painful and cause infections and swelling. Round or oval nails are not suited to the toes as the nails rub against shoes.

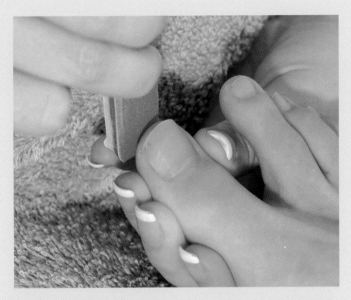

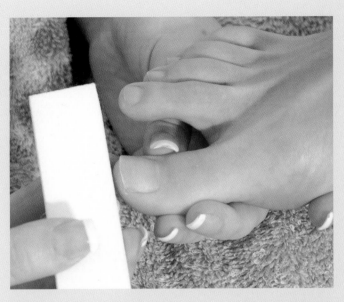

⑦ Once you have shaped the toenails, bevel them to remove any rough edges which could interfere with a smooth varnish application. Bevelling is practised by turning the nail file to 90 degrees and filing straight down on the free edge where rough nail edges can lie.

⑧ Buff the nails with a block or three-way buffer to bring about a natural shine. Often toenails develop ridges over time and so the buffing action will smooth the nails' appearance and allow the varnish to lie evenly on the nails.

⑧ Apply a small amount of exfoliating scrub and massage into the feet and legs for about 5 minutes. This will smooth out the skin and remove any dead skin cells before starting the massage, making the skin more receptive to the essential oils that will be applied. Once the scrub has been rinsed off, pat the skin dry. It is important to make sure you are comfortable before starting the massage to gain the maximum effect from it.

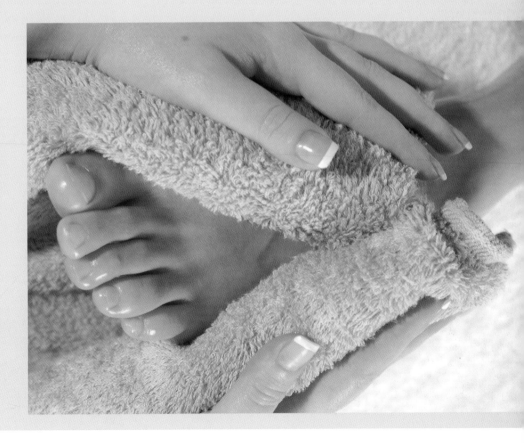

FOOT MASSAGE ROUTINE

Warm the foot moisturiser or oil in your hands first, then apply to the feet and follow the routine outlined here.

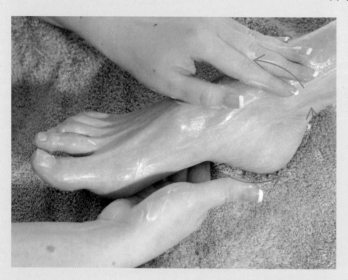

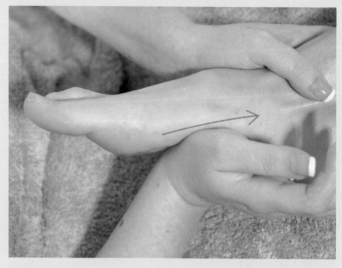

① Working on one foot at a time, rub the foot to ensure it is warm before you start. This increases circulation and the depth of pressure you can apply during the massage by making the foot muscles more flexible. Rub the moisturiser or oil onto the foot. Holding the foot, rotate the ankle to increase joint flexibility in the tarsal bones.

② Using the heel of your hand massage up and down the sole to awaken the reflexology points and to soothe the arch of the foot. You may feel small nodules of tension. If this is the case concentrate on these to release the tension in the muscles.

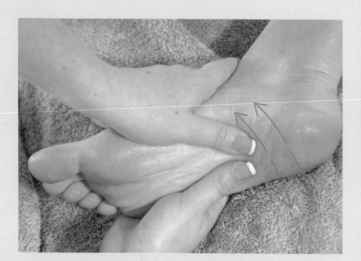

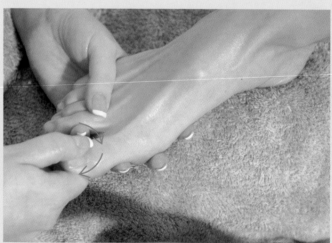

③ Using small thumb circles work from the heel to the toes and deeply massage the whole of the sole.

④ Rotate each toe to increase flexibility and massage the cuticle area to stimulate growth from the matrix.

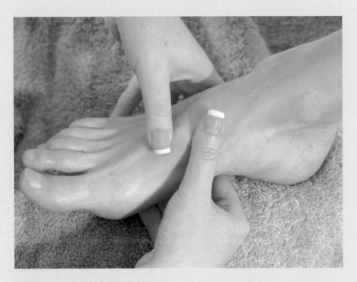

⑤ Thumb knead the top of the foot to increase circulation. Apply slightly less pressure here as you are directly working on superficial veins which do not require such heavy stimulation.

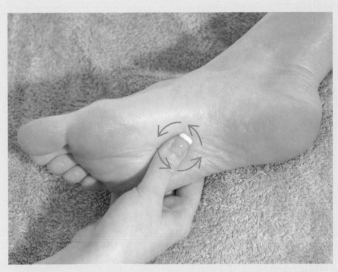

⑥ Slowly and deeply massage the solar plexus point on the foot, which is found just below the ball. This area represents the centre of your body and internal wellbeing.

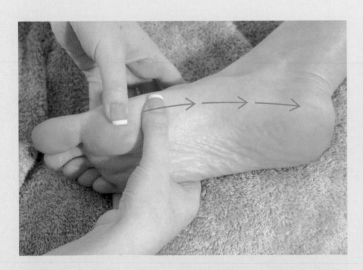

⑦ Massage deeply over the spinal reflexes which run from the heel to the big toe. Do this three times whilst taking deep breaths.

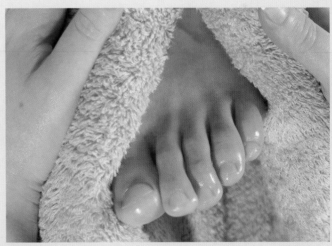

⑧ Hold the foot and warm it before wrapping it in a towel and proceeding with the massage on the other foot.

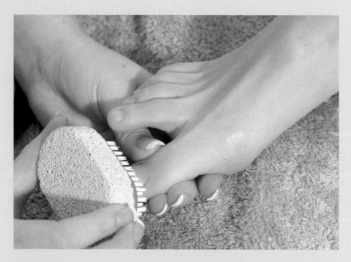

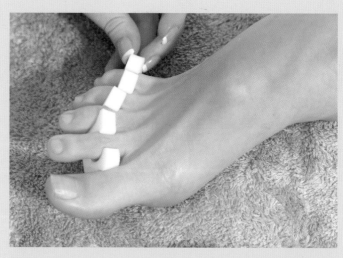

⑨ After the massage brush over the toes with a nail brush and some warm water to remove all traces of oil.

⑩ Pat dry and prepare to varnish by inserting toe separators. Apply a base coat to the nails to prevent the varnish from staining the nail plate and leave to dry. Apply two coats of varnish, being sure not to flood the cuticle area or the nail wall.

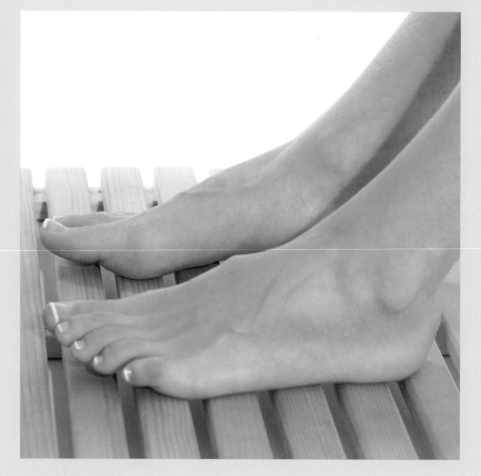

⑪ Finally apply a top coat to secure and protect the finish. Allow the varnish to dry thoroughly for about 20 minutes before putting on shoes. To help the nails dry quicker, pool a little cuticle oil on the surface of the varnished nails to provide a protective layer. This works really well and could be the difference between a smudge nightmare and a smooth finish.

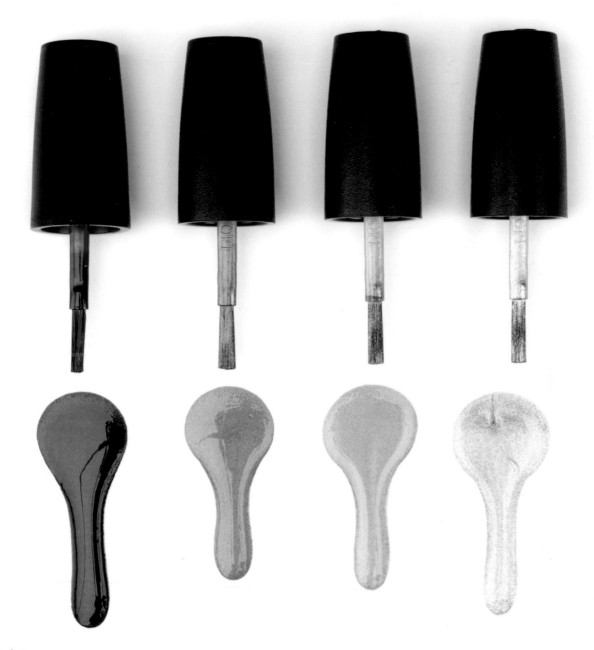

Varnishing

Toenails, too, have types and some will be very hard and brittle whereas others will be weak and difficult to grow. Treat them the same as finger nails and apply a base coat that contains a nourishing treatment to balance the nails. This does not mean buying a separate nail treatment for fingers and toes, just use the same one!

Ensure the consistency of the varnish is smooth and not too gloopy. Choose a colour you like or one that matches your outfit. This type of accessorising is really impressive and looks great!

For the best application of varnish load one side of the brush with varnish and ensure the neck of the brush is clean of dripping colour. Try to apply the varnish in three strokes and as quickly as possible, making sure no colour goes on the cuticle or nail wall area. To make nails look longer apply the varnish on the nail leaving a slightly wider gap all round the sides of the nails and apply close to the cuticle area. This gives the impression the nails are longer and slimmer than they actually are!

Once happy with your colour choice lock in the colour and protect it with a layer of shiny top coat which sets hard to provide a coat of protection.

how to...

FRENCH PEDICURE

Celebrities favour the French pedicure look, so much so that toenail extensions can now be applied to feet in the French style! Before attempting a French pedicure ensure a full pedicure has been performed as it is important that the nails are clean and free from dead surface cells and any natural oils. This helps the polish last longer and go on smoother.

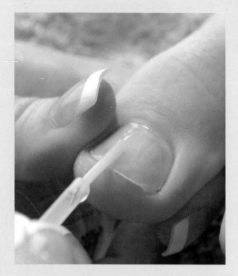

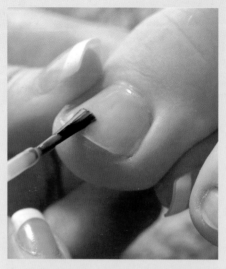

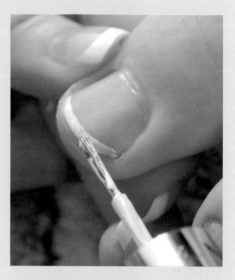

① Start by applying a protective base coat (toenails can go yellow very easily even with a light-pigmented varnish).

② For the best and most dramatic look apply one or two coats of the pink base, depending on your preference.

③ Finally stroke on the white tips either with the help of pre-cut paper stencils or freehand.

④ Allow the varnish to dry for as long as possible, preferably overnight, and when choosing which pink or white base to use go for the pinkest pink or the whitest white! Anything too creamy in colour will fade into your natural nail colour and be less noticeable. After all your hard work you will certainly want people to see the results!

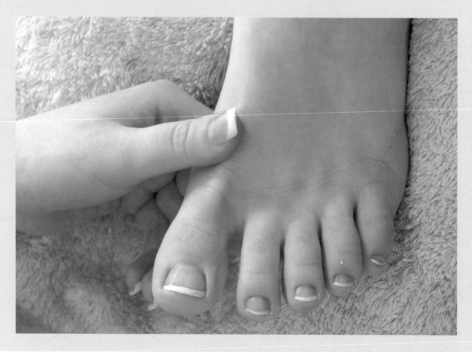

Professional therapy

Professional treatments are widely available these days in nail bars. Pedicures tend to be a little more expensive than manicures so expect to pay extra. Treatments such as hot stone therapy, paraffin wax, hot oil therapy, masks, thermal booties and salt spa treatments are all designed to add to your pampering session.

Feet respond to hot and cold substances and both energise the cardiovascular system and make it work hard to balance the body's temperature. This tried and tested method of improving circulation has been used for centuries in Sweden where people run from hot saunas to roll in the snow! Heat is always nicer but both extremes in temperature have a part to play in improving circulation and mobilising joints. It is important to recognise that looking after your feet pays off. The occasional pampering is well worth it!

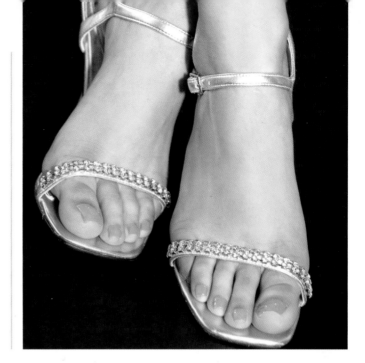

how to...

FOOT MASKS

Masks on the feet are generally applied to nourish dry skin and to cool and revitalise tired and puffy feet. Don't apply a foot mask over open wounds or sore skin as this will irritate the skin and can be painful.

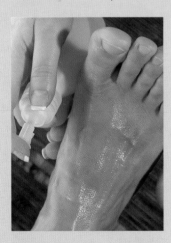

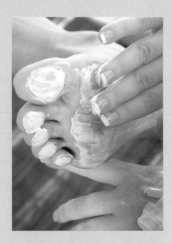

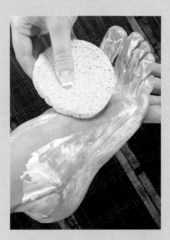

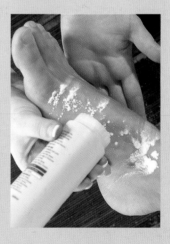

① **Firstly, clean the feet and if applying a mask as part of a pedicure, do it just after the massage.**

② **Apply the mask on the soles first as these require longer treatment, and then the tops of the feet to the ankle and lower legs. Raise the feet and wrap them in a towel to keep them warm.**

③ **Rest for 10 minutes and remove the mask by soaking the feet in a foot spa and sponging off.**

④ **It is important to moisturise after the mask as absorbent clays can dry the skin. Alternatively apply foot powder to maintain dryness whilst deodorising feet.**

Skin scrubs

That feeling of silky smooth feet is just fantastic and the appearance of soft clean feet is very seductive! Foot scrubs come in the form of creams, gels or even mitts with rough exteriors to scrub off dead skin cells. Coarse sea salt can also be a great exfoliator and will absorb excess sweat from the skin, too.

If doing a pedicure at home, scrub your feet after using a rasp or pumice for the best effect and really rub in the product for around 10 minutes to really slough off all remaining skin cells. Rinse and pat dry to remove the scrub, then proceed to the rest of the pedicure. Often scrubs and masks go really well together, especially in the summer, leaving your feet feeling cool, zingy and refreshed.

Warm wax

As covered in The manicure (see page 73), paraffin wax has been used for many years to help warm and soften the skin on the feet. It can also encourage mobility in the bones of the ankle (tarsal) and toes (phalanges), which can induce relaxation. The feet are susceptible to dryness, especially around the heel and so it is even more important to apply a thick layer of wax to the soles and then the tops of the feet. A cream under the wax will boost the moisture content and the heat will allow the skin to absorb the oils found in the wax more effectively, leaving your feet warm and smooth.

Warm wax and oil treatments are great in the winter but can be a refreshing change in the summer months, too. Hot oil is used all year round to deeply nourish the skin on the feet and to prevent cracked heels and splitting nails.

how to...

SKIN SCRUB

Exfoliation is key to maintaining soft, silky skin, especially on areas that are prone to dryness and hard skin, like the feet. Concentrate on the soles but work all over to achieve a smooth all-over finish.

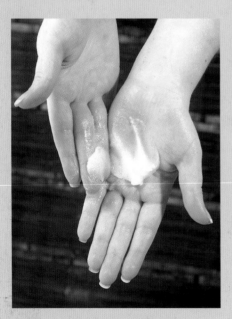 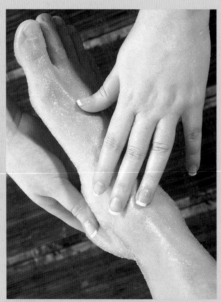 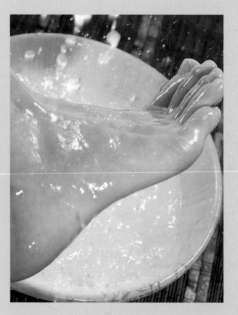

① **After cleaning the feet apply a walnut-size amount of scrub to the hands and rub together to warm.**

② **Apply in circular movements and vigorously rub around the feet, especially the ankles and lower legs, for around 10 minutes.**

③ **Soak the feet to remove the scrub granules and pat dry before proceeding with the rest of the pedicure.**

how to...

WARM WAX

The most pampering treatment of all, this is a must for anyone with dry skin or chapped heels.

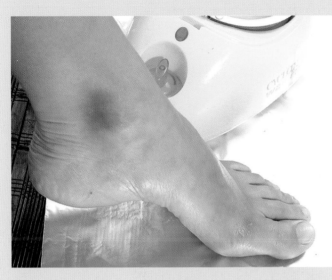

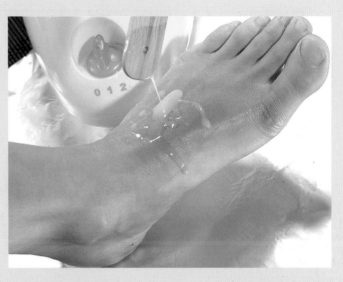

① Place the foot on a plastic bag or tin foil to prevent the wax from dripping onto any surfaces.

② Ensure the wax is not too hot by testing it on the inside of your wrist first. Brush on or drizzle the warmed wax over the area, remembering to apply it to the underside of the foot first, especially around the heel.

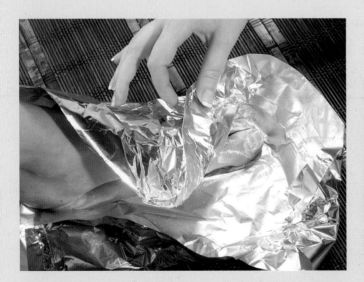

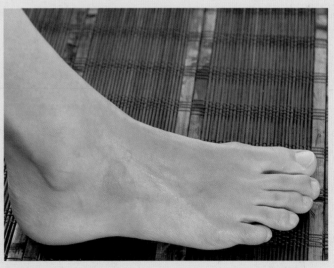

③ Wrap up the waxed area in the foil or plastic and then a towel for 10 minutes.

④ Unwrap the area and pull away the wax easily to reveal super soft, warm feet!

how to...

HOT OILS

Bones, muscles and the circulatory system crave warmth, and hot oil treatments combined with massage are difficult to beat. Warm a small bowl of almond or grape seed oil over a larger bowl of just boiled water, then apply the warmed oil to the feet for a soothing, relaxing treat.

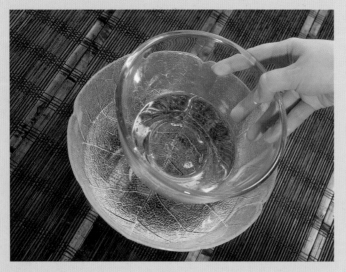

① **Warm a small bowl of oil over a larger bowl of hot water for a few minutes.**

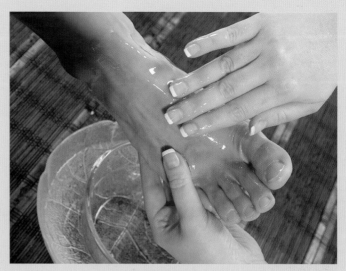

② **Apply the warm oil to the feet and massage in to keep the feet warm and increase mobility to the joints.**

③ **Wrap the feet in plastic or foil to retain the heat and relax for 10 minutes while the oil is being absorbed and softens harder skin tissue.**

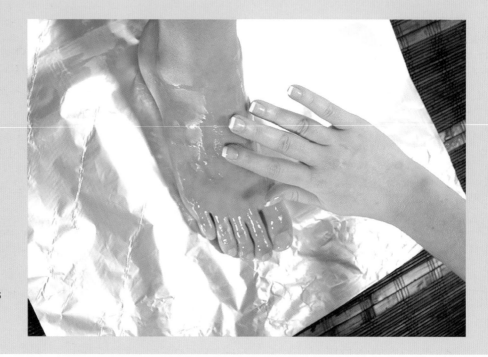

The professional pedicure

Having a pedicure is a must for anyone contemplating wearing flip flops or sandals. It is also an amazing experience and often people treat the nail bar as a social event, going with friends for a chat and gossip! The treatment itself will not be all that different to the home treatment described earlier. Feet are hard to reach so let a nail technician take over and allow yourself to really be pampered. Pedicures are almost as popular as manicures and often clients book them in simultaneously to save time.

Expect a high standard of hygiene, clean tools and a qualified and well presented nail technician. Your therapist should do a thorough consultation to assess your needs and diagnose your nail and skin types which will help in picking specific treatments for you. It is vital for your nail technician to know what you want. I always let my technician know what varnish I would like and if I think my nails are too weak or if they split easily. Your nail technician should always apply a treatment to your nails and not just a base coat.

The nail industry is renowned for employing minimum wage technicians who work on commission so they will be very keen for your return business. This battle for clients also inevitably cuts the price of treatments, so if you have received good service and you can afford to, you may wish to leave a tip. This will imprint your name and face on the technician's memory and they may fit you in next time when they are normally busy!

The male pedicure

The male pedicure is exactly the same as the female pedicure, except for the varnish stage as most men will not want a coloured polished finish! Quite often men have better looked-after feet because they never wear high heels of pointy shoes. Looking after feet decreases the risk of corns, joint pain and ingrown toenails. Men often like to have a coat of nail treatment to complete the pedicure but rarely is this a shiny varnish. It is worth investing in a male matt base to coat the nails as this will protect them as well as treat the nail type.

Male feet can look nice and taking time to treat yourself to a pedicure is really worthwhile. If you play a lot of sport you may find your nails are bruised or black due to the constant pressure they are under from trainers and sports footwear. This can be difficult to rectify but seeking the advice of a specialised footwear company may help to diminish the chances of unsightly toes!

NAIL BAR DO'S AND DON'TS

✓ Do expect good service. There are so many nail bars your technician should be fighting for your custom.

✓ Do expect your pedicure to include at least all the steps you would do in a home treatment: soak, cuticle work, exfoliation, massage, filing and varnish.

✓ Do feel free to talk to your technician and ask questions about what products they are using on your feet and which are the best to use at home.

✓ Do expect to see notice of insurance visibly in the salon.

✓ Do expect to feel relaxed after a pedicure. You should not come away feeling stressed!

✓ Do expect your nail technician to be knowledgeable. He/she should be properly qualified, trained and insured.

✗ Don't leave unhappy. Always make a point of giving constructive feedback as this can only improve the service. A little knowledge goes a long way so if you know something is wrong, then mention it politely.

✗ Don't sit in pain if your technician is too heavy handed. Ask them to be gentle to ensure your treatment is more comfortable.

✗ Don't have a pedicure when the foot spa has not be cleaned or the water changed. Dirty tools and equipment will lead to cross infection of diseases and skin disorders so insist on good hygiene practices or seek treatment elsewhere.

✗ Don't expect your pedicure to dry instantly. Be organised by bringing flip flops with you. Your nail technician will have to move onto their next client so be prepared to dry in the waiting area or flip flop away!

how to...

EXFOLIATION AND PEDICURE

Pedicure treatments make feet feel soft and smooth but also help to relax muscles.

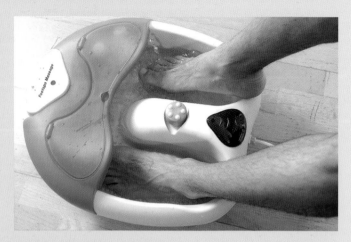

① Fill a foot spa or foot bath with warm water and soak the feet for 5 minutes. For added benefit, add a handful of coarse sea salt, a teaspoon of milk and three drops of essential oil of peppermint, eucalyptus or sandlewood to create a fresh and balancing environment.

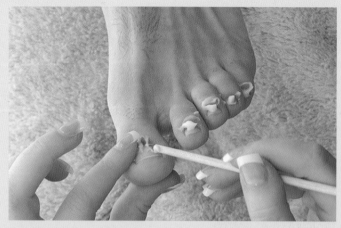

② Apply a pea size amount of cuticle cream to the cuticles and rub in. This emolient cream will make cuticle removal easier. Place the feet in the spa for a further 2 minutes, then pat dry.

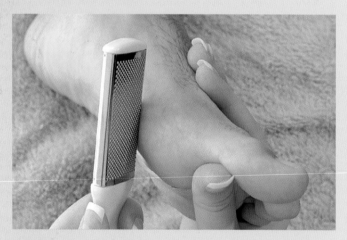

③ Use a metal foot rasp to gently remove the hard skin from the heels, toes and balls of the feet. Do not rub too hard and keep checking the area until you can no longer feel the build up of hard skin. The rasp will make rough skin disappear quickly but will also leave the skin feeling slightly uneven so even out the skin by buffing it to a smooth finish. Use the fine foot buff or pumice to smooth the skin's surface.

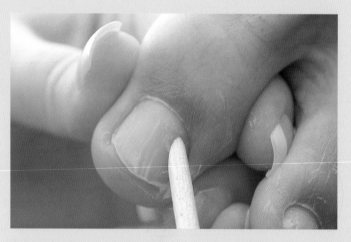

④ Push back the cuticles and remove any surface cuticle cells from the nail plate using a cuticle knife or orange wood stick.

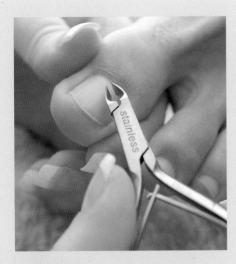

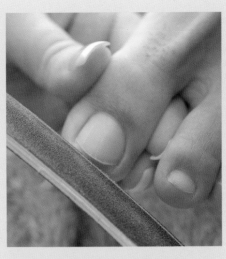

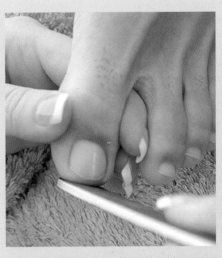

⑤ Excess cuticles may need to be trimmed off with cuticle nippers but be sure to leave a little amount to protect the matrix from damage.

⑥ Trim the free edge and file it into shape. The best shape for toenails is square as it keeps the nails from in-growing. Avoid cutting nails too short as this can encourage ingrowth. Leaving them too long may increase the chance of a bruised toe during sporting activities or excessive walking.

⑦ Now bevel the nails to remove any fluffy bits which could interfere with a smooth treatment application. Bevelling is practised by turning the nail file to 90 degrees and filing straight down on the freed edge where fluffy bits of nail can lie and need to be removed.

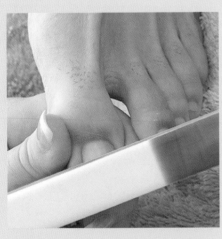

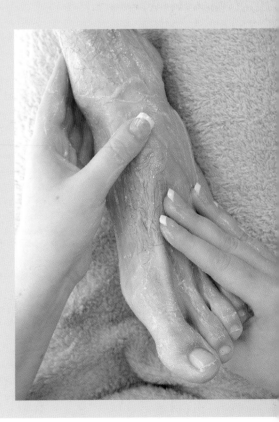

⑧ Buff the nails with a block or three-way buffer and bring about a nice natural shine.

⑨ Apply a small amount of exfoliating scrub and massage into the feet and lower legs for about 5 minutes. This will smooth out the skin and remove any dead skin cells before the massage making the skin more receptive to the essential oils that will be applied. Once the scrub has been rinsed off, pat the skin dry.

MASSAGE ROUTINE

Warm the foot moisturiser or oil in your hands first, then apply to the feet and follow the routine outlined here.

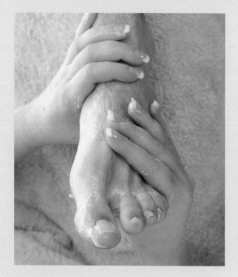

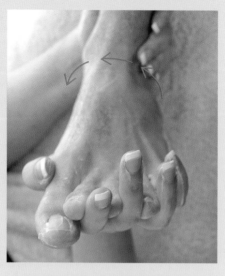

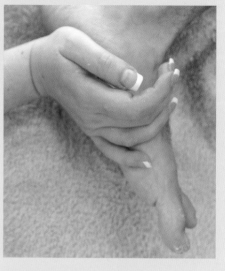

① Rub the feet to warm them, then rub in the oil. This increase in circulation maximises the depth of pressure you can apply during your massage.

② Holding the foot, rotate the ankle to increase joint flexibility in the tarsal bones.

③ Using the heel of your hand, massage up and down the sole to awaken the reflexology points and to sooth the arch of the foot.

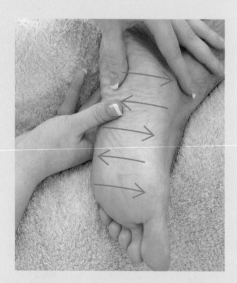

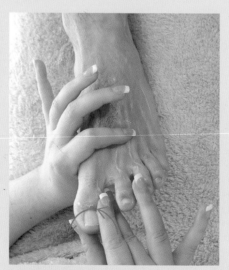

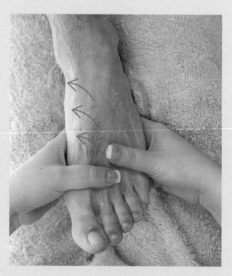

④ Using small thumb circles, work from the heel of the foot to the toes and deeply massage the whole of the sole.

⑤ Taking each toe in turn, rotate it to increase flexibility and massage the cuticle area to stimulate growth from the matrix.

⑥ Thumb knead the top of the foot to increase circulation.

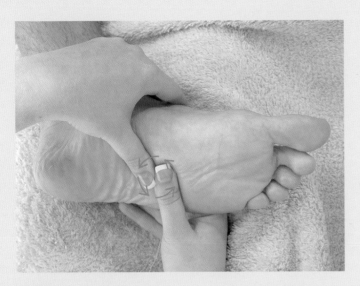

⑦ Slowly and deeply massage the solar plexus point on the foot, which is found in the middle of the foot just below the ball.

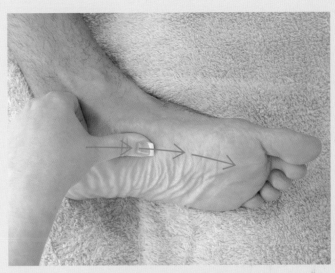

⑧ Massage deeply over the spinal reflexes, which run from the heel to the big toe, three times whilst taking deep breaths. Hold the foot and warm it before wrapping it in a towel and proceeding with the massage on the other foot.

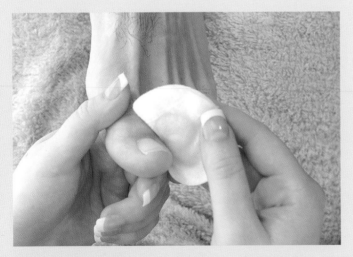

⑨ After the massage wipe over the toes with a varnish remover and some warm water to remove all traces of oil, which could impair the adhesiveness of the base coat. Pat dry and prepare to apply a protective treatment to the nails.

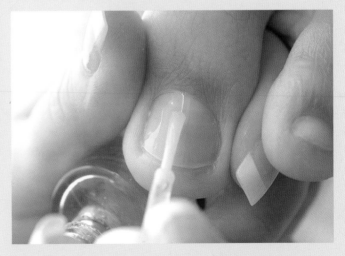

⑩ Apply a base coat or specific nail treatment to the nails to protect the nails and allow to dry thoroughly before putting on socks and/or shoes.

Artificial toenails

Artificial nails have only recently been used on toes to improve the general appearance of the nails and to give natural nails more growing power. All the usual methods of applying artificial nails are suited to the toes and the results are perfect. All three systems of acrylic, gel and fibreglass or silk are very popular on toes, with acrylic being the preferred choice as it is the hardest wearing substance and will sustain the pressure from shoes.

ACRYLIC

Acrylic is by far the most popular system to use on toenails as it is strong, durable and easy to refill as the nail grows out. The possibilities are endless with acrylic but the most popular look is that of the French pedicure which can be achieved with coloured acrylic alone. This saves time with varnishing the toes, and the nails will always look the same.

Once plastic nail tips have been applied for added length the acrylic mixture of powder and liquid is applied to coat and form the nail itself. Acrylic is quick, strong and looks natural if applied properly. The downsides are that it is smelly, messy and the acrylic is often so hard that any bangs to the nails can result in tremendous pain! These are long-lasting nails and need filling every two to three weeks. Removing them requires melting the acrylic with acetone which takes a while and is costly so do not have acrylic nails for a one night wear. You are looking at three to six weeks minimum.

There are three ways of applying acrylic to the nails: on top of a nail extension, applied to your own natural toenail to add strength, or applied to the free edge of your toenail to add length and then over the whole nail for strength.

Whichever method you choose there are a few golden rules to remember when using acrylic:

The application of an acrylic nail in theory is relatively simple, in practice however it is hard to do very well! Do be patient with acrylic and master the art, especially on the toes, as it really is a specialist treatment so being good at it will make you in demand!

THE TOOLS FOR ACRYLIC

① 100/180 grit file
② Cuticle oil
③ Extension clippers
④ Cotton wool discs
⑤ Block buffer
⑥ Acrylic powders
⑦ Orange wood stick
⑧ Acrylic brush
⑨ Extension form

▽ *This basic tool kit is used for both manicures and pedicures.*

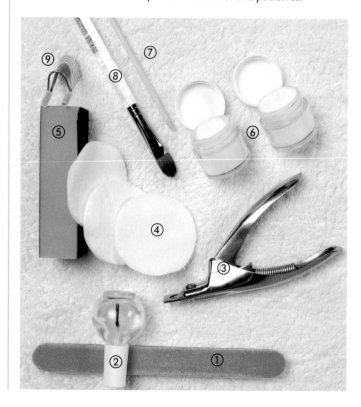

how to...

ACRYLIC TOENAIL EXTENSIONS

Acrylic is tough, durable and easy to maintain – so easy that you could have a French pedicure all year round!

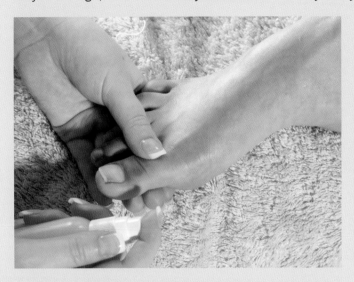

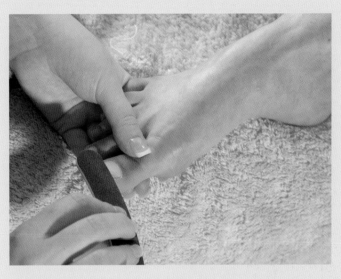

① Clean the toenails of varnish and sanitise them thoroughly. If the cuticles are long push them back now.

② File the natural nails down to prolong the life of the extensions. Bevel to remove any fluffy edges after filing or block buff.

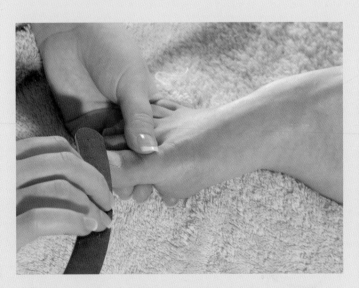

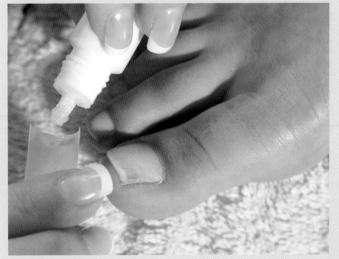

③ Scuff the whole surface of the nails with the finer side of the nail file. The nail plate is very thin so if it feels hot, then you have filed too much away.

④ When all the nail plates are rough and dull, size your extension tips to the size of the nails. Apply the tip after filling the lower edge of the tip with adhesive nail glue. With very light pressure and ensuring no air bubbles have formed under the surface of the tip, place and push the tip onto the nail just below the free edge.

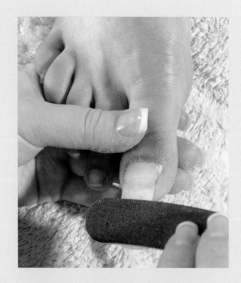

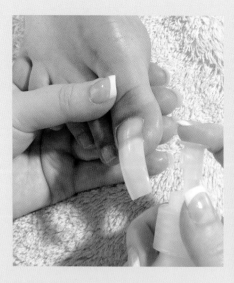

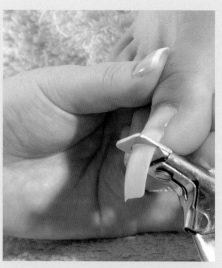

⑤ File across the base of the plastic extension until there is no visible line between the extension and the natural nail. Effectively you have blended the appearance of the two together.

⑥ To ensure a sterile environment spray the nails regularly with antibacterial spray which will neutralise bacteria but evaporate quickly, leaving you with a clean working surface.

⑦ Cut the length you do not require off the extension and shape the end of the extension to suit your needs. A square shape is best and the perfect length for toenails is the length of the toe itself. So file just to the end of the toe flesh and not below.

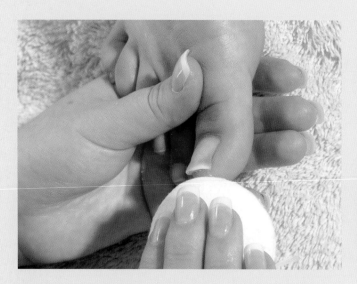

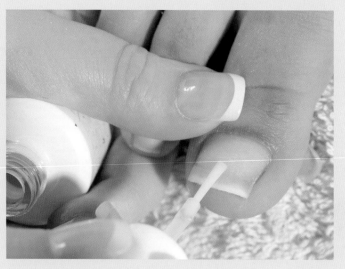

⑧ Remove the excess nail dust by brushing with a large nail brush, then wipe the plates with varnish remover to ensure they are clean of debris that would otherwise affect the application of acrylic.

⑨ Dot nail primer (methacrylic acid) onto the nails. This is an irritant substance which aids the attachment of acrylic to the nails. Be sure not to get it on the skin as it will sting; although no damage will be done it can feel uncomfortable.

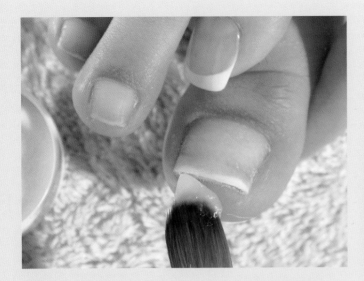

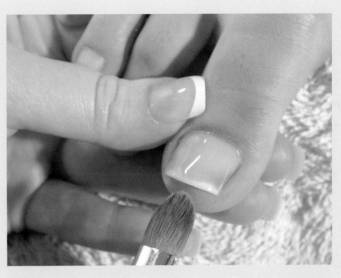

⑩ Hold the toenail firmly and with the other hand dip the brush into the acrylic liquid. Once it is saturated remove the excess by pressing it to the side of the glass dish and dip the tip of the brush into the acrylic powder. Once the powder is wet you have about 20 seconds to mould the acrylic before it starts to harden, so you will need to work quickly.

⑪ Apply a small ball to the tip of the toenail where the joint from the tip was before you blended it with the file. Place the second ball close to the cuticle and smooth over the whole nail. Repeat this move with the third ball and finish with a ball on the tip again but brush backwards from tip to cuticle. The acrylic can be manipulated but allowing it to run a little down the nail can help you apply a smooth coat.

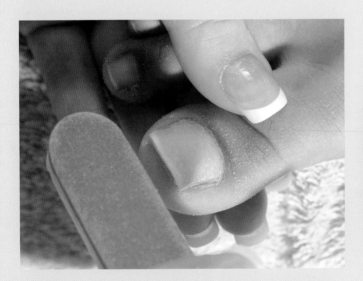

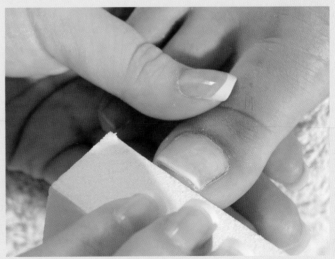

⑫ Allow the acrylic to dry for 30 seconds and tap until you hear a click sound which implies it is totally set. Using the 100/180 grit boomerang, buff the roughness of the nails all over and refile the free edge if necessary.

⑬ After the nail plate is smooth and there are no visible gaps or joins, work the block buffer over the nails, refining the surface of the acrylic until it is completely smooth. Apply a little cuticle oil and allow to absorb for a few minutes before washing the feet thoroughly. Once the feet are clean and dry apply the varnish of your choice and top coat to seal the colour.

GEL

The gel system produces the most natural looking finish as the gel substance is completely transparent. It is known as a pre-mixed system because there is nothing to mix: the gel is just one substance which is set with UV light.

Nail gels do not harden in the presence of oxygen and so the extra UV light is required to act as the catalyst to allow the gel to harden. Most gels leave a slightly sticky surface after drying but if this is wiped away correctly it is not a problem. Some gels are very thin in consistency and these are best used as top layers due to their shiny appearance or to build up thin layers on natural nails for extra strength. Thicker gels carry more strength and are better for use with extensions.

The preparation for gel nails is virtually the same as acrylic but the overall effect is more natural but less hardwearing so depending on your needs you can choose a system to suit you.

THE TOOLS FOR GEL

1. **100/180 boomerang grit file**
2. **Cuticle oil**
3. **Block buffer**
4. **Gel brush**
5. **Crystal nail file**
6. **Gel**
7. **Cotton wool discs**
8. **Extension clippers**

▽ *Equipment for gel nails can be expensive but they are worth it and last a long time. Keep them clean and tidy to maintain hygiene.*

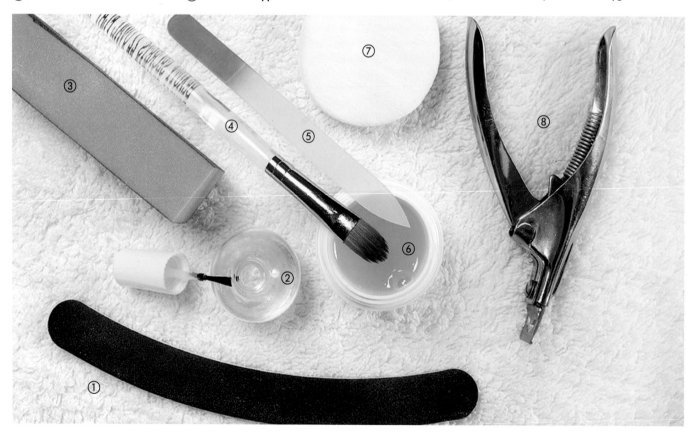

how to...

GEL TOENAIL EXTENSIONS

Gel extensions are the most natural looking of the three systems, so on the feet gel works out to be great option.

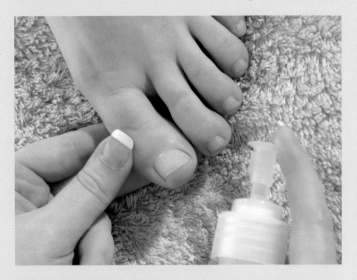

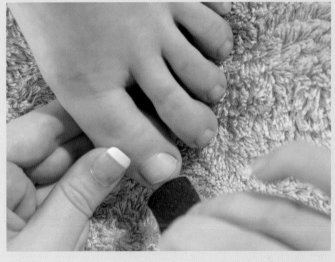

① Clean the toenails of varnish and sanitise them thoroughly to ensure there are no bacteria lying on the surface of the nails. If the cuticles are long push them back.

② File down the natural toenails to prolong the life of the extensions. Bevel to remove any fluffy edges after filing or block buff.

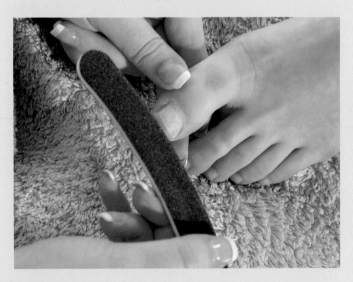

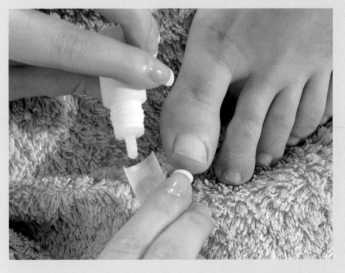

③ Scuff the surface of the nails with the finer side of the nail file.

④ Once the nail plates are rough and dull, size your extension tips to the fingers ensuring they are an exact match by filing excess tip away. Apply the tip after filling the lower edge with adhesive nail glue. With light pressure and ensuring no air bubbles have formed under the surface of the tip, place and push the tip onto the nail just below the free edge.

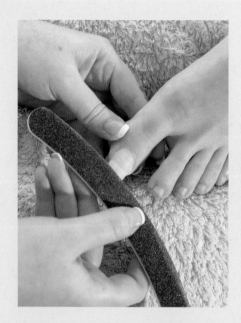

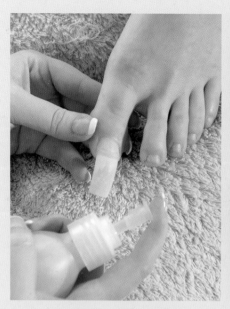

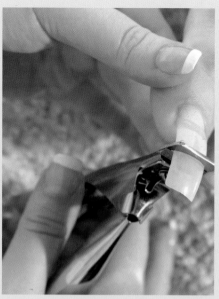

⑤ File across the base of the plastic extension until there is no visible line between the extension and the natural nail.

⑥ Spray the nails regularly with antibacterial spray to neutralise bacteria, leaving you with a clean working surface.

⑦ Cut the length you do not require off the extension and shape the end of the extension nail to suit your needs. Square is the best option for toenails.

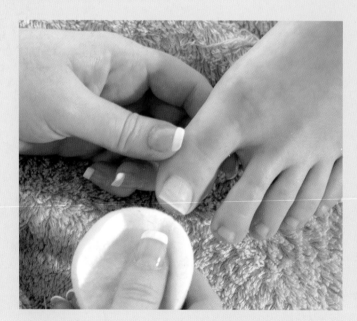

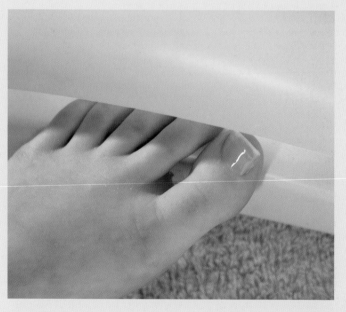

⑧ Remove the excess nail dust by brushing with a large nail brush and then wipe the plates with varnish remover to ensure they are clean of debris that could affect the gel application.

⑨ Switch on the UV light and start applying the gel to all toes of one foot only. A thin coat will do as a base, just be sure not to get any gel on the skin. Place the toes under the light for 2 minutes while you repeat on the other foot.

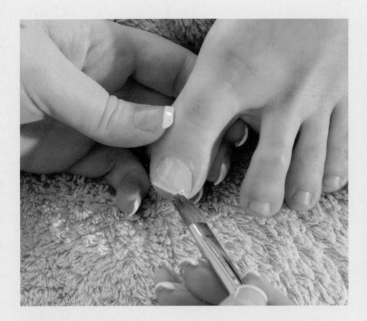

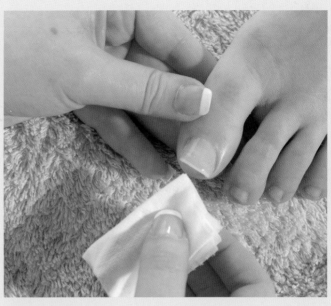

⑩ Repeat the application three times so each toenail has three layers of gel. Place the toes under the UV light after every application to cure each layer independently.

⑪ There may be a sticky residue on the nails after the final curing under the lamp. Gently wipe this away with a nail cloth.

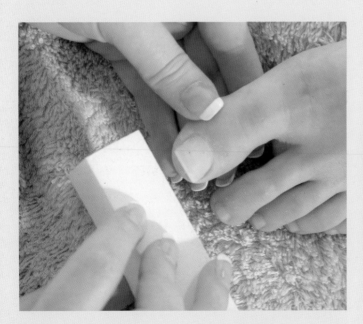

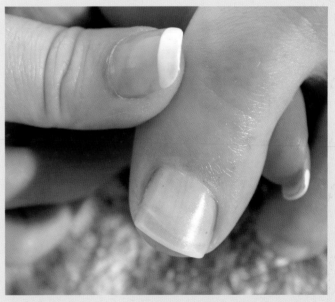

⑫ Using a nail file or buffer, smooth the surface of the nails until they are smooth and buff to a high shine.

⑬ Apply cuticle oil to the skin to re-nourish and wash the feet to clean away all debris. Leave the nails as they are with a top coat or varnish with your choice of colour to finish. Apply a top coat to increase the durability of the colour.

FIBREGLASS AND SILK

Developed by beauty therapists the fibreglass and silk systems were born after a stronger alternative to glue and tissue paper was needed for mending nail breaks and splits. The three-component system of fibreglass or silk mesh, resin and resin activator allows the nail technician to build up natural nails layer on layer to provide a strong and sturdy extension.

Personal preference will indicate whether you use silk or fibreglass, but both are very strong. The mesh is sticky on one side so it can be easily applied to the nail in a strip from cuticle to tip. Fibreglass is slightly more durable but does not turn clear when dampened by the resin whereas silk is almost totally clear and becomes one with the resin so can look more natural. The resin used is a chemical of the acrylic family but it will dry and harden when exposed to air alone. Ethyl cyanoacrylate is a popular choice of nail companies for resin and it is used in many industries as a reliable adhesive for wood, metal and piping!

Activator spray is used to speed up the process of hardening the resin (naturally it takes about 15 minutes to harden). The activator cuts this time down to a few seconds but if applied incorrectly it can be very uncomfortable and burn. The spray must be applied from a 30 cm (12 in) distance as if too close the skin can feel like it is burning or irritated. Along with this uncomfortable reaction the resin will crack and produce a weak overlay with many tiny cracks in it.

THE TOOLS FOR FIBREGLASS AND SILK

① Block buffer
② Fibreglass/silk sheets
③ Cotton wool discs
④ Cuticle oil
⑤ Extension clippers
⑥ 3-way final polish buffer

▽ *Fibreglass and silk tools are not only great for nail extensions but also double up as a nail repair kit.*

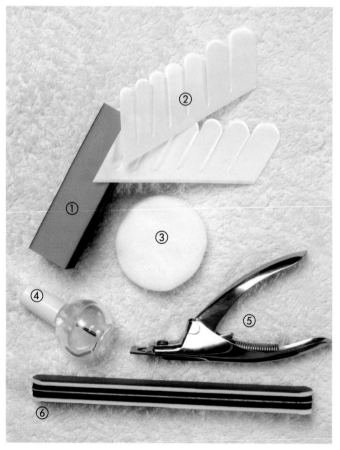

trade secrets

- To ensure the mesh cannot be seen through the resin make sure you wet the mesh thoroughly on the first application otherwise the end result will be unnatural and the mesh very visible.

- When applying the mesh leave a little gap around the edge of the whole nail as this will provide a much more natural look to the nail when finished.

- Do not over buff as the resin may be filed away quickly and expose the precious mesh which will look terrible and often the nail will have to be done again.

- Do not breath in or get resin or activator in your eye as it will sting and medical attention will be needed immediately.

- When applying resin try to ensure each layer is of a medium density. Layers that are too thick or too thin weaken the strength of the extension.

how to...

FIBREGLASS AND SILK TOENAIL EXTENSIONS

Fibreglass and silk can provide extra strength to real toenails or extensions. Apply more resin to the big toes but ensure all toes have an even coverage of resin.

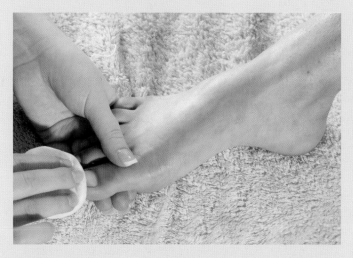

① Clean the toenails of varnish and sanitise them thoroughly to ensure there is no bacteria lying on the surface of the nail. If the cuticles are long push them back now.

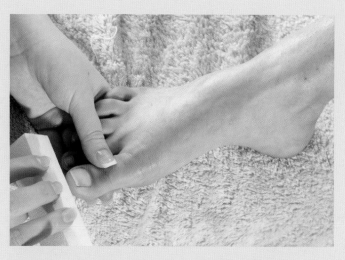

② File the natural nails down to prolong the life of the extensions. Bevel to remove any fluffy edges after filing or block buff.

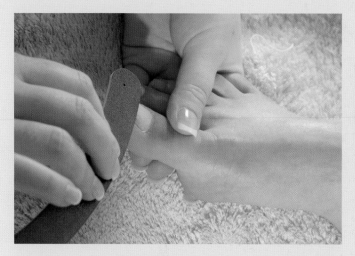

③ Scuff the surface of the nails with the finer side of the nail file being careful to lightly cover the plate.

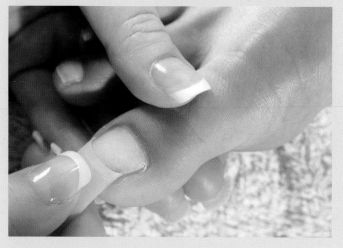

④ Once all the nail plates are rough and dull size your extension tips to the fingers ensuring they are an exact match by filing excess tip away. Apply the tip after filling the lower edge of the nail with adhesive nail glue. Place and push the tip onto the nail just below the free edge.

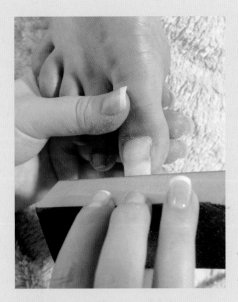

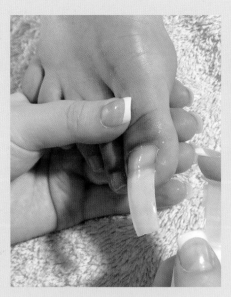

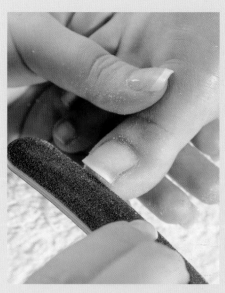

⑤ **File across the base of the plastic extension until there is no noticeable line between the extension and the natural nail.**

⑥ **Spray the nails regularly with antibacterial spray which will neutralise bacteria and leave you with a clean working surface.**

⑦ **Cut the length you do not require off the extension and shape the end of the shorter nail to suit your needs, again square is the best choice for toenails.**

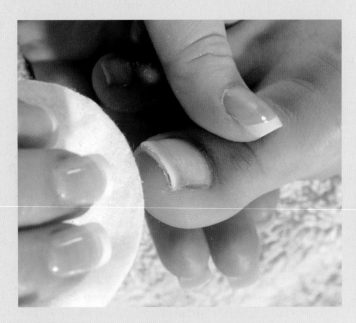

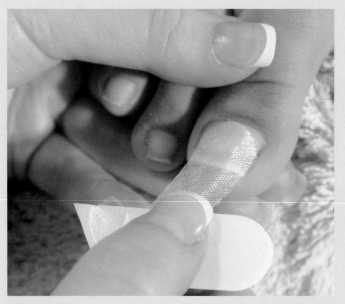

⑧ **Remove the excess nail dust from the nail by firstly brushing with a large nail brush and then wipe the plates with varnish remover to ensure they are clean of debris that could effect the resin application.**

⑨ **Apply the mesh to the nail with the sticky side on the nail plate, leaving a small gap round the sides and cuticle of the nail. Pre-cut fibres are now available which speeds up the process as no cutting and shaping is required.**

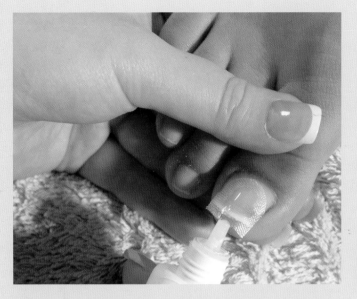

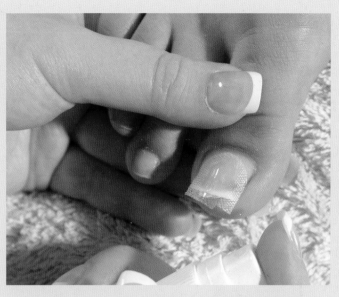

⑩ Cut the excess mesh and wet with the first layer of resin. Spray at 30 cm (12 in) to activate the resin when you are sure it is all wet and has turned transparent. Make sure there in no resin on the skin before spraying as this will feel like burning.

⑪ Apply the second coat of resin and spray followed by a third and final coat of resin and spray to activate. If the nozzle clogs replace it or try a brush-on product it you find them easier.

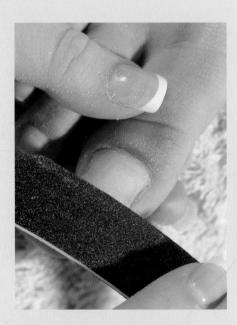

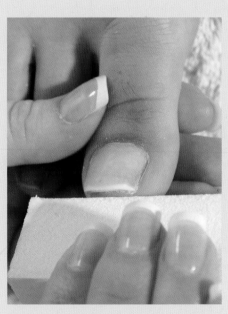

⑫ Once the three coats are dry file lightly to remove unevenness with the nail file and block buff with the buffer to smooth and complete the treatment.

⑬ Varnish to finish or buff to a shine if you prefer the natural look.

AND LASTLY...

Acetone in a small bowl will remove acrylic and fibreglass nails by breaking down the bond of chemicals which make it and melting them off. However gel nails are not easily removed by soaking and will simply require buffing off. Be careful whilst doing this as the nail can become hot and tender so go slowly and have regular breaks for the nail to cool.

Never pick or leaver off nail extensions of overlays as the damage to your natural nail will be extreme. Always soak where you can and the nails will not be as damaged.

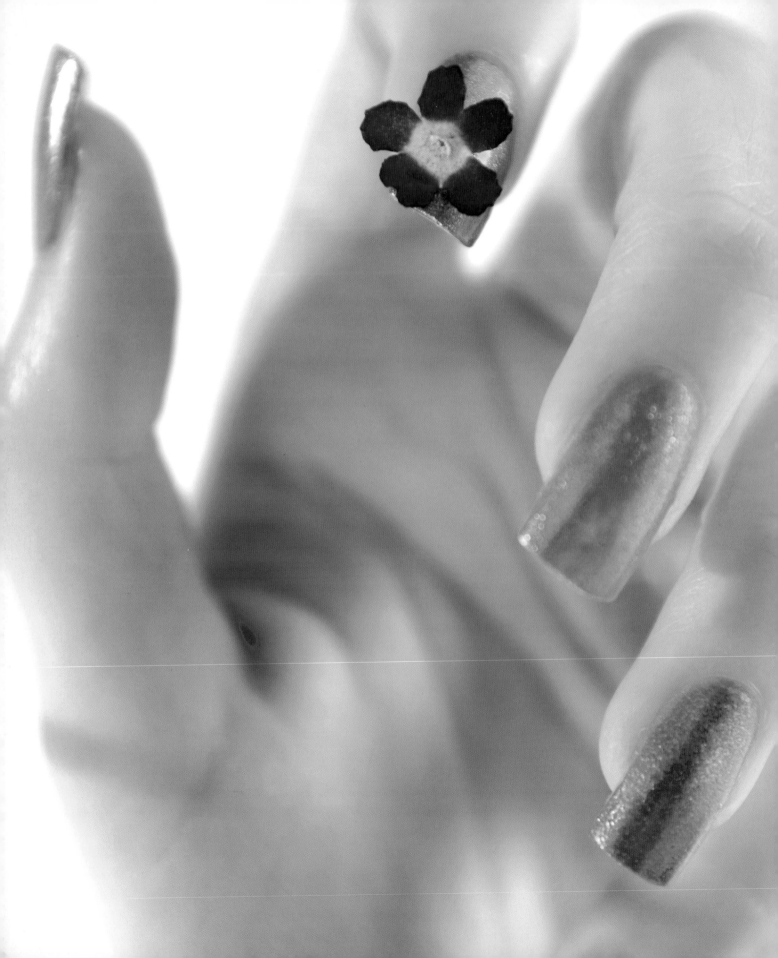

09 the art

the art

Ever since the ancient times when blood was mixed with animal fat to colour the nails we have strived to make nails look beautiful. People will always have differing ideas as to what beauty is and some of the nail designs featured here are wild and outrageous whereas others are simple and stylish – the choice is yours.

Plain varnish can be just as eye-catching as bright patterns or sparkly designs on nails but depending on the desired effect choose a design you won't mind wearing for more than a few days!

Nail varnishes

Nail colours and varnishes vary hugely and there are many textures and styles to choose from:

Matt This no-shimmer finish is very popular with the professional woman. Whether in dark or pastel colours the idea of a matt finish is both understated and elegant.

Gloss This shiny finish varnish is stunning. Gloss varnish is very popular especially in highly coloured or dark varnishes as the visual effect is glamorous.

Pearlised The varnish of choice for older women, this varnish rarely needs an extra top coat and has a shimmery, pearly finish to it.

Glitter Glitter varnishes look terrific for an evening look. A touch of glitter added on top of any varnish creates a glitzy finish.

Metallic These copper, gold or silver varnishes block out the nail completely and look very dramatic whether the nails are short or long.

Glow These clever varnishes glow in the dark! Some even change with your body temperature so it looks as though you have several colours on during the evening, depending on how hot you get!

Mood changing As with glow varnish, these varnishes change colour according to the temperature of the nail bed. They can look very effective as the nails will have a two-tone appearance.

With polish alone there is a huge choice of textures, colours and finishes, but nail art doesn't stop there by a long way. Whether you have natural or artificial nails, jewellery, stones, glitter, drawings and stencils can all be placed on the nails to create amazing designs that will make your nails truly individual! If you can dream it you can put it on a nail – from a beach scene or a whale to your favourite flower or your own personal design!

▷ *Wear a varnish that mirrors your emotions.*

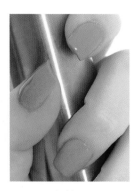
△ *Matt*

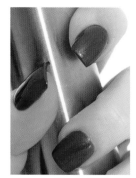
△ *Gloss*

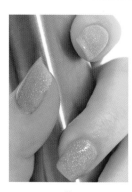
△ *Glitter*

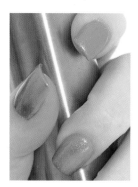
△ *Metallic*

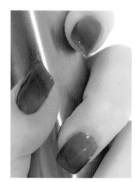
△ *Mood changing*

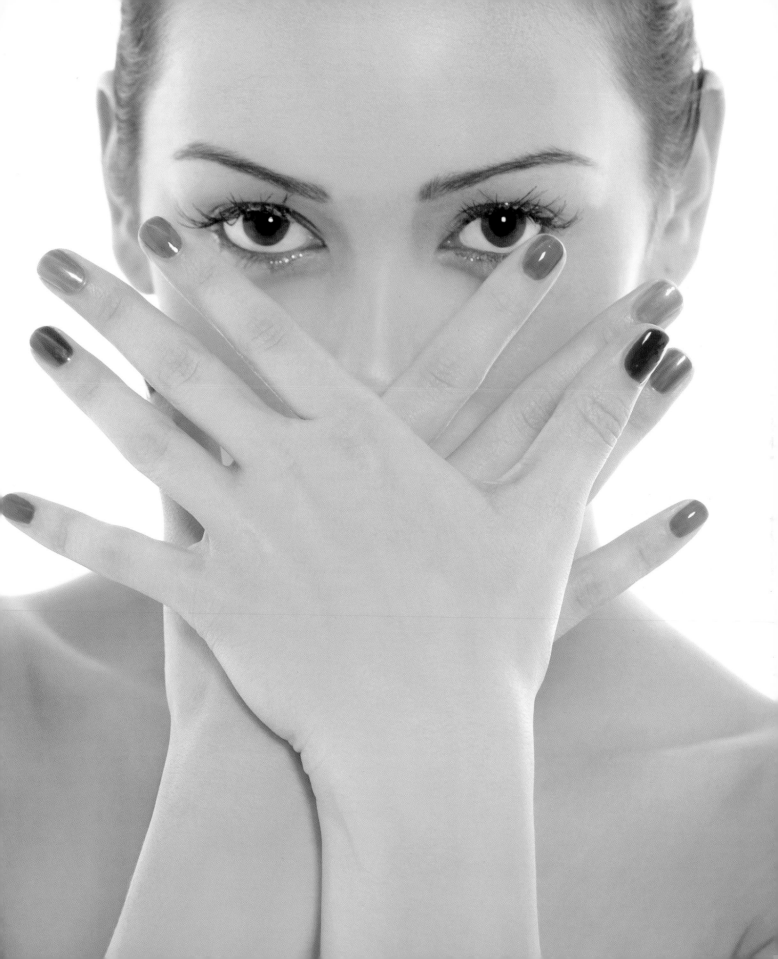

Design tools

Nail design is a form of art and like all arts, it needs the right tools. The nail art palette includes the following implements:

Varnishes Coloured and clear varnishes, along with top and base coats.

Acrylic-based coloured paints These non toxic paints can be used for all painting work as well as airbrushing.

Brushes Usually a fine brush is used for drawing straight lines, a fan brush for feathery designs and a tiny straight brush for dots and precision work.

Transfers The best to buy are the water-release ones as they are easily applied and are not as bulky as the self-adhesive ones.

Embossing tool This syringe-like tool is used mainly to create raised dots but the marbling attachment at the other end of the tool can also create an embossed effect.

Tweezers These are essential for guiding artwork into place as fingers are often too warm and bulky for this intricate work.

Orange wood stick This is a handy tool for sticking and detaching nail art so one in your art box will always be useful.

Nail glue Can help to stick difficult transfers and other nail art pictures.

Glitter, rhinestones, crystals, jewellery, stencils and stick-ons Are all options and can be useful when you are feeling creative to produce a dazzling picture but leave them out if they are not your style!

① **Transfers and stick-on art**   ④ **Foil**
② **Glitter and rhinestones**   ⑤ **Fan brush**
③ **Shiny metallic strip paper**

▽ *Nail art tools come in many forms and if you like nail art, try everything!*

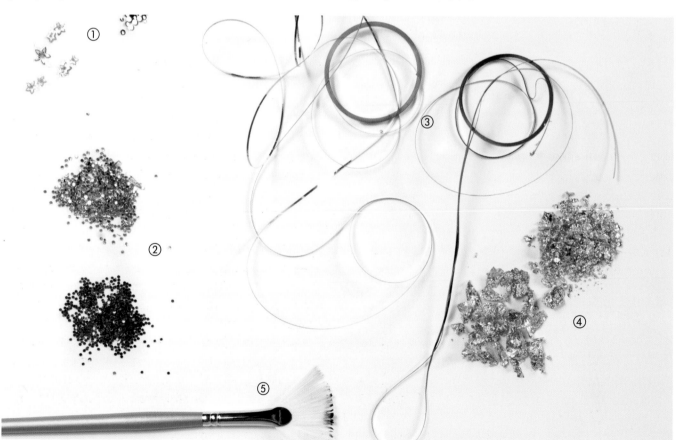

Artistic answers

There are many ways of creating nail effects and designs on nails, and often the best method is to airbrush on patterns and designs. In this modern industry of nail art any shape or design can be achieved – even a photograph can be printed onto nails! There are a few things you can do at home to jazz up your nails and they are simple techniques anyone can do.

RHINESTONES AND GLITZ

Rhinestones come in many colours and sizes and allow for vast imaginations, from simple designs to elaborate compositions! Suitable for all ages, these can bring a smile to the face of every onlooker.

Apply a colour to the nails if you wish, then apply a base coat over the top to make the nails sticky. Whilst the base coat is still wet work quickly to place the stones in the design of your choice using tweezers or an orange wood stick for greater accuracy. Complete with a top coat to secure your artwork.

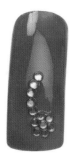 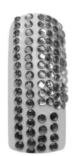 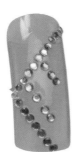

FOIL LEAF [insert 4669]

Gold, silver, copper or platinum foils for the nails are stunning when used subtly on the nails. Foils are easy to apply and can add a touch of individuality to nails.

Tear small chunks of foil off the main sheet and apply to a wet coat of base. Use an orange wood stick to apply and secure in place wherever you desire.

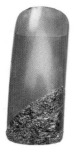 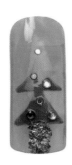 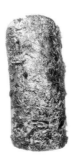

STRIPES AND STICK-ON NAIL ART

Strips of coloured sticky tape help to create defined lines on the nails for flag and box designs. They can be coloured in or act as a dividing line between matt varnish and shimmer, but whichever way you use them they could not be more simple to apply.

Ensure the nail varnish base colour is completely dry, then apply the strips of coloured tape to the nails using tweezers to position them. Always over estimate the length of the tape and measure it exactly from the cuticle or nail wall first. Trim the excess and finish with a top coat to super secure your design.

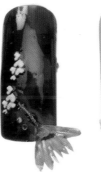 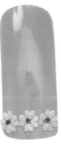 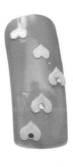

NAIL DESIGN TRANSFERS

These designs are mounted onto clear film just like any other transfer and are just as easy to apply. They are long lasting, especially with a clear top coat to finish.

Check the transfer fits the nail perfectly and place it upside down on the nail. Dampen a cotton bud and wipe it over the transfer. Once the transfer changes colour or turns transparent gently press your thumb onto the transfer and it will stick to the nail. A top coat will secure any design but if you wish to add to your design do so before applying the top coat.

GLITTER AND GLOSS

Glitter is a great way of instantly drawing attention to the nails and creating a really wild effect. Glitter comes in many forms but often the pure dust variety is just as good as paper or large particle glitter.

Start by applying a coat of varnish or a base coat. Once you have chosen your design and while the varnish or base coat is still wet, dip the tip of the brush into the base coat and then into some glitter to create a ball. Apply and spread the ball to fit your design! Once the glitter has dried apply a top coat to seal and protect the nail art.

EMBOSSED DESIGNS

Embossing is performed by using a metal drip (embossing) tool or a plain plunger dispenser which acts like a syringe and as the plunger is pressed the paint comes out the fine tip like a ball.

Ensuring your tools are clean, map the design with the tool to ensure it fits onto the nail. Emboss the design onto the nail and wait at least 20 minutes for it to dry before top coating twice to prevent chipping.

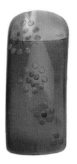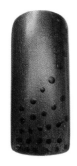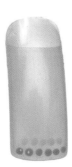

MARBLING

This look is great to show off your nail art talents! Marbling is generally applied with vivid colours but also looks nice with pale or dark colours.

Using the metal embossing tool, apply drips of different colours down the centre of the nail. After they are all on the nail use the tool to swirl the paints together to create a curly, marble effect. A top coat seals the art and protects it from chipping.

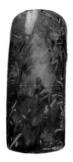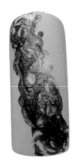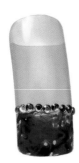

FREEHAND DRAWING

Often considered the hardest nail art to perform as this requires a steady hand and some great imagination! Drawing any design needs preparation but if clients have a picture or a stencil to work from it can be easier. Often just one or two showcase nails will have freehand work but for a special occasion why not have them all done!

BRUSH STROKES

This looks great for a party feel and because it looks random it carries a carefree theme to your nails.

Apply a white base coat and then one colour on top of another until you are happy with the look of the nail. Brush on the colour horizontally across the nail to give a windswept look. Finish the design with a top coat and dry.

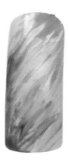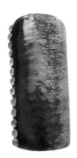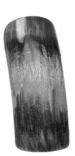

Nail jewellery

Nail jewellery is increasing in popularity. Nail piercing is now very common with finger rings, studs and even clip-on jewellery available for an eccentric look.

Nail piercing tools are inexpensive and this type of added accessory can be very effective! Just be sure not to go over the top otherwise the effect can be spoilt.

A tiny hand-held screw will drill a hole in the nail and the jewellery is either clipped on or attached through this hole. Rings and studs can be attached this way, too, but the more elaborate the jewellery the heavier it is so be aware that nail extensions are usually strong enough to carry the extra weight on your nail tips but natural nails may break under the pressure.

All types of nail art can also be used on toenails and can be extremely effective. Because toenails are seen from a distance use bold designs so that the detail can be seen and your hard work can be appreciated and admired!

Often people tend to opt for darker colours as they are more noticeable but a classic French pedicure or some simple gems can be just as effective. With a pedicure extension you could utilise jewellery or more elaborate foot jewellery but be careful about wearing close-toe shoes as the constant rubbing could lead to nails breaking or splitting which can be painful.

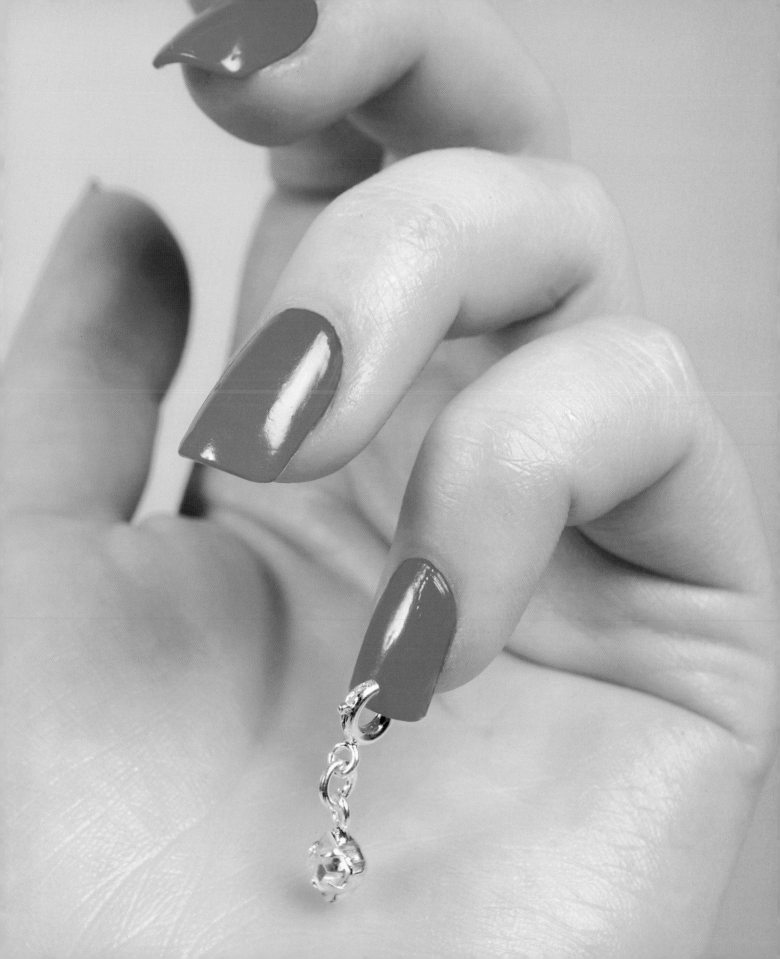

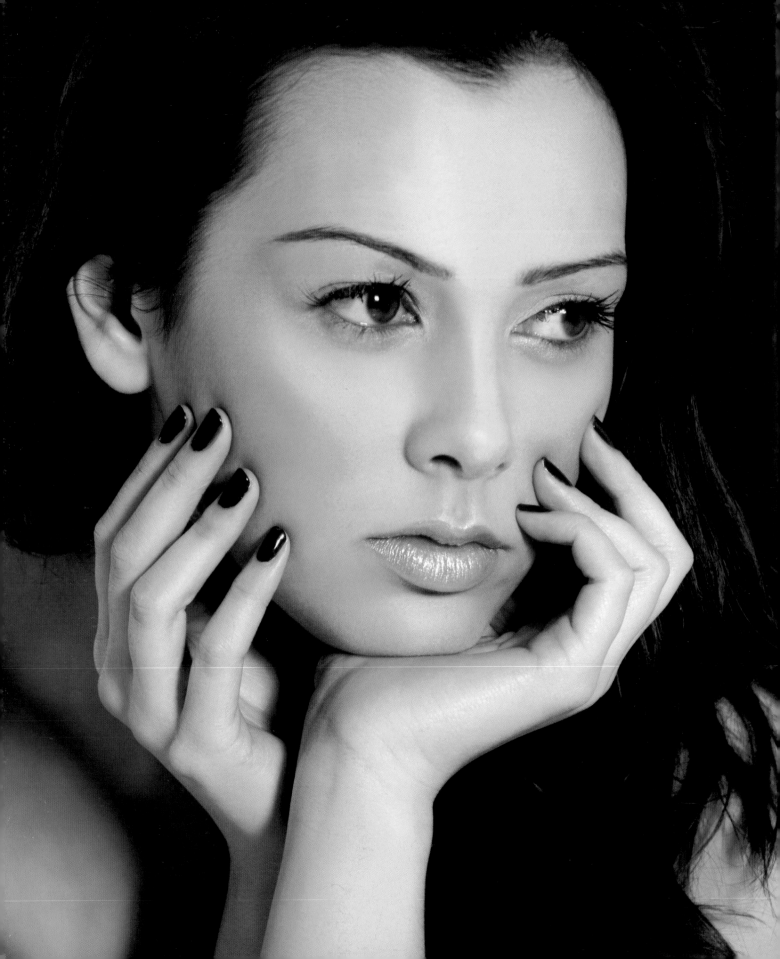

10 the looks

the looks

Finger and toenails can make or break an image! Some icons past and present have been known to wear particular nail colours. This chapter illustrates some of the most popular looks of decades past and present so you can try them out for yourself.

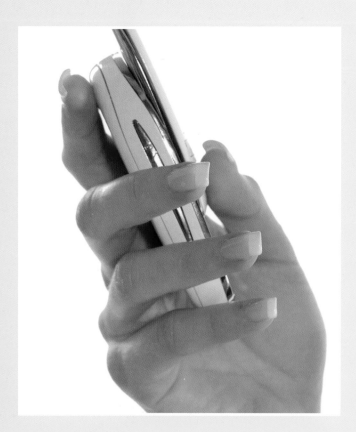

◁ French fancy

The French finish to nails is a classic choice and leaves the nails looking clean, fresh and well groomed! It can be done on short or long nails and on hands and feet. Whether your nails are shaped round, oval or square, this crisp, clean look is very popular and will always be a favourite with young professional women.

see pages 144–145

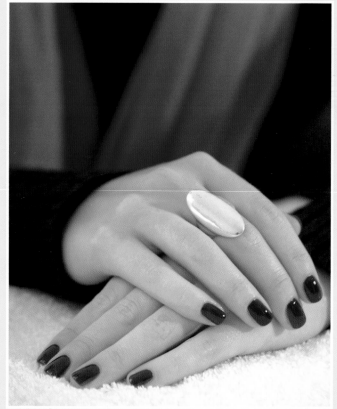

▷ The vamp

This very popular vamp look is great for anyone who really wants to show off their nails to the full. Ensure you have a square finish to relatively short nails for maximum impact and pre-manicure or pedicure to ensure the nails are at their optimum. This colour suits everyone but avoid going very dark on varnishes if you have mature hands as paler colours will complement you fabulously.

see pages 146–147

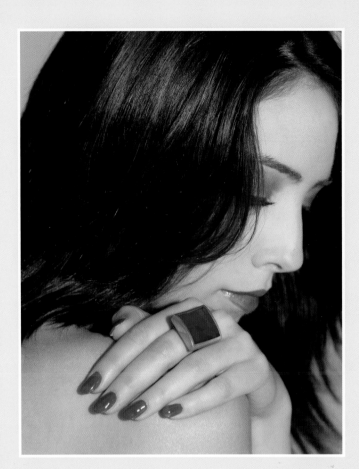

◁ ravishing red

Red has always been a popular colour on nails but can look bloodthirsty on some skin tones. It is best suited to olive skins.

see pages 148–149

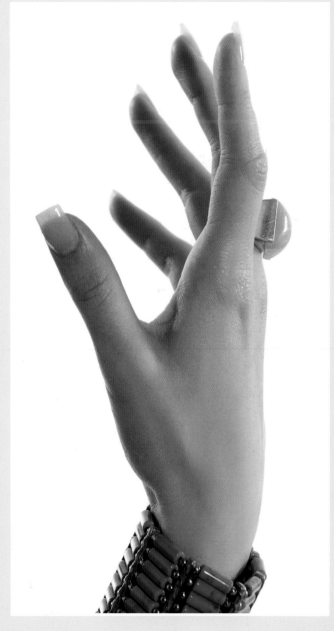

▷ nearly naked

Often the best nails are those that look naturally beautiful. We all desire perfect looking nails that look like we've never done a day's work in your life. These can be achieved – even if you do work hard!

see pages 150–151

how to...

CREATE THE FRENCH FANCY LOOK

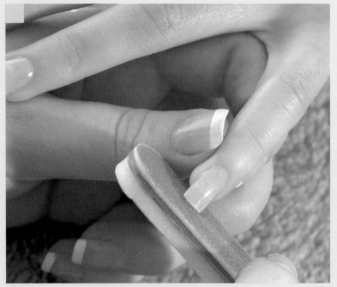

① Ensure you complete a full manicure or pedicure treatment to smooth and soften the skin and shape the nails to a square finish.

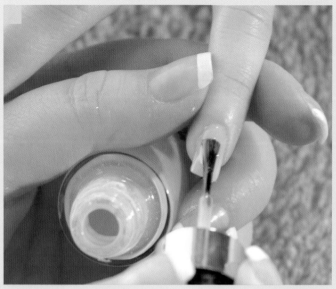

② Apply two coats of French pink on top of the base coat and allow to dry.

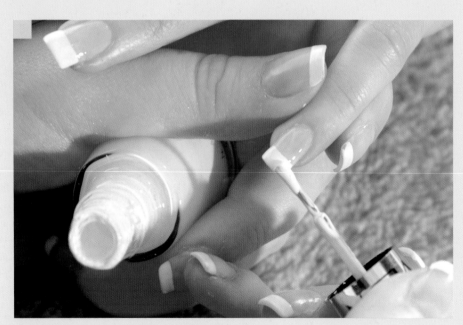

③ Apply two coats of white varnish to the tips of the nails or free edge. You can make nails look longer by exaggerating this white line.

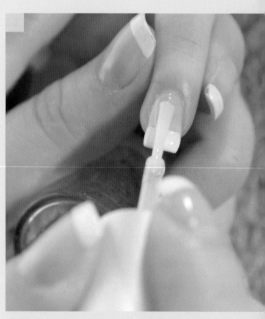

④ Finish with a thick layer of top coat to seal. If you wish, add a fine line of glitter in between the two colours for an extra glamorous look.

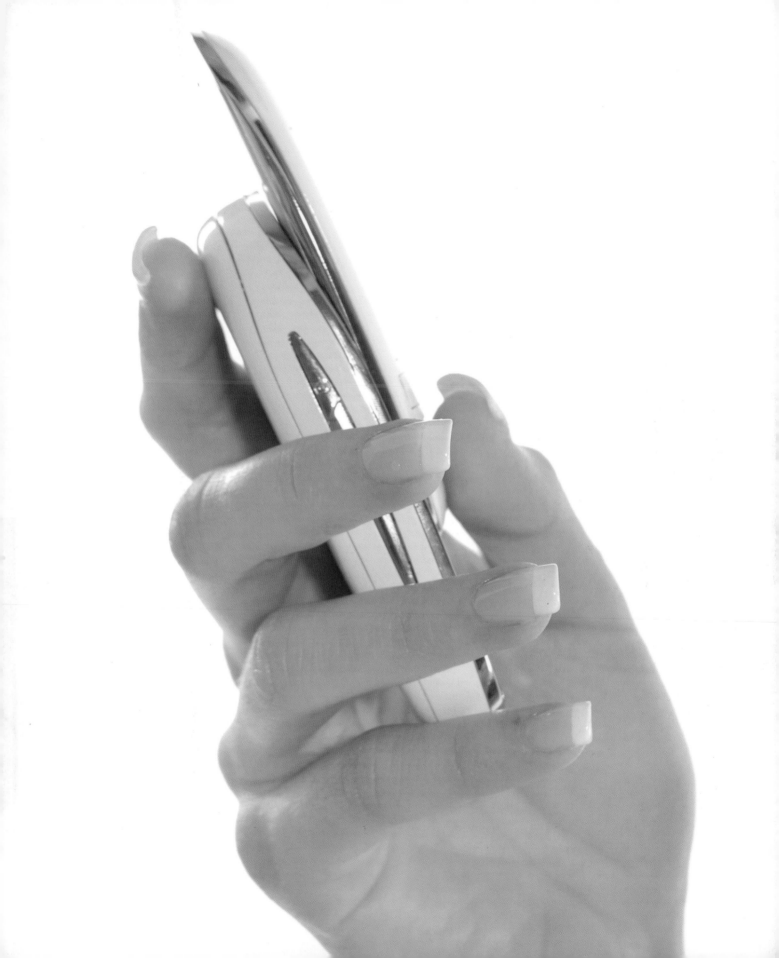

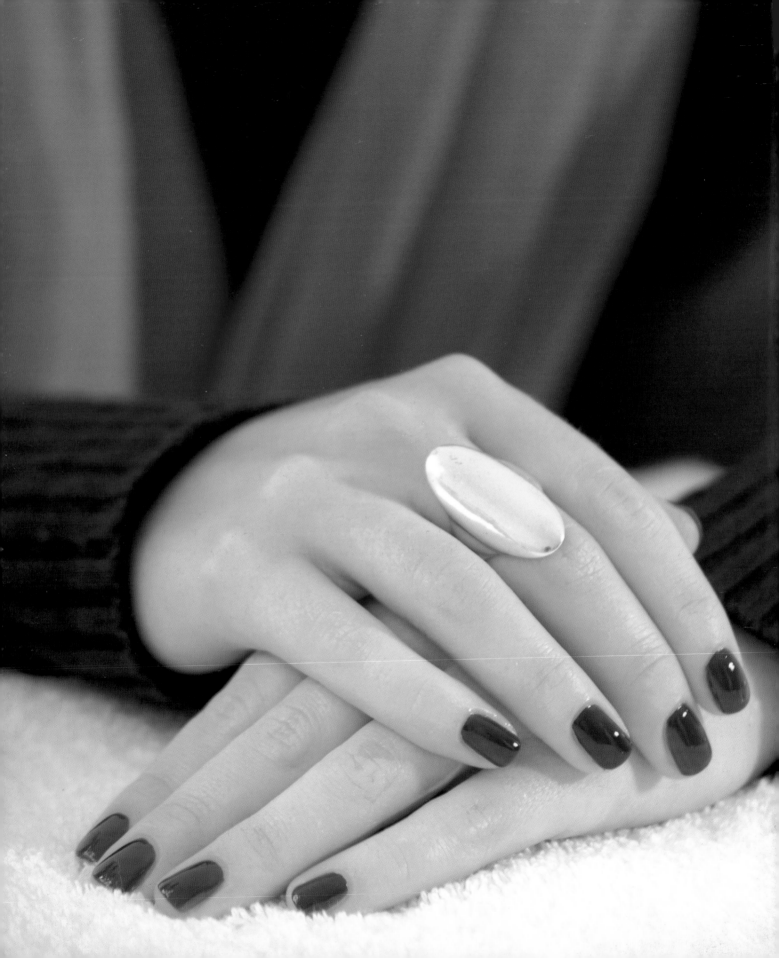

how to...

CREATE THE VAMP LOOK

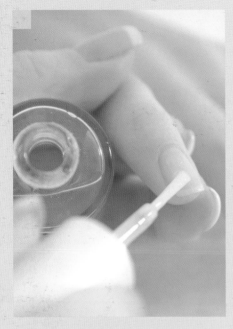

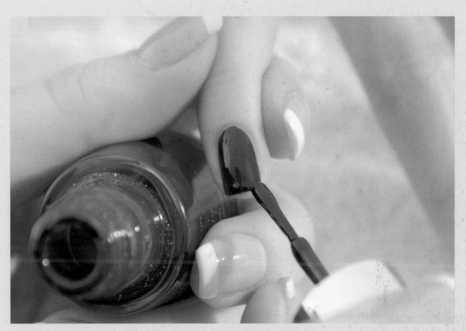

① Apply a base coat to the nails and allow to dry completely. The pigment in this varnish is very dark so a heavy base is best to protect the natural nails from discolouring.

② Apply two generous coats of dark plum, smoke or black to the nails. Be sure to take your time with dark colours as any small slip or shake takes time to correct with varnish remover! Beginners should leave a thin unvarnished line around the base and sides of the nail to protect the cuticle and nail wall from spillages. As your varnishing techniques improve, reduce this space until the varnish meets the cuticle and nail wall perfectly with just a fraction of a millimetre to spare.

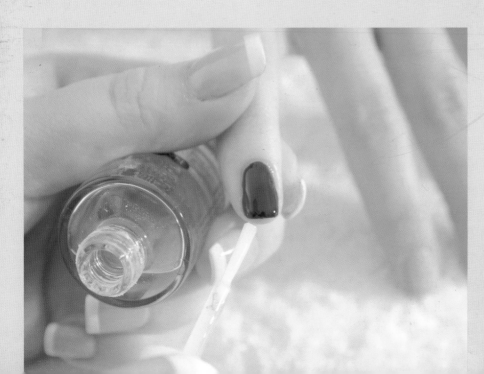

③ Finish with a high gloss top coat and allow to dry to give an ultra shiny finish to the varnish. Top coat also prolongs the life of coloured varnish and keeps it looking fresher for longer.

how to...

CREATE THE RAVISHING RED LOOK

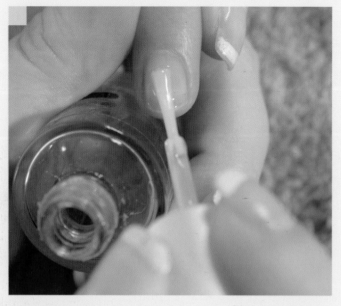

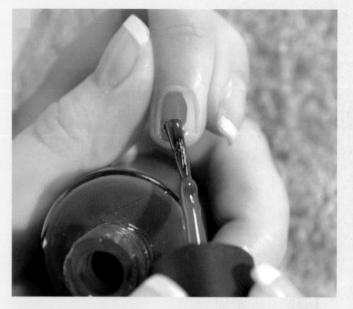

① Apply a base coat to the nails and allow to dry completely to prevent the varnish running into the cuticle area. Drying should only take a matter of minutes so patience is rewarded with a much smoother surface for the colour to adhere to.

② Apply two thick coats of red varnish. Be careful not to get varnish in the cuticle or nail wall area as this could look like you have cut your finger! Be careful and go slow in order to achieve this fabulous classic look.

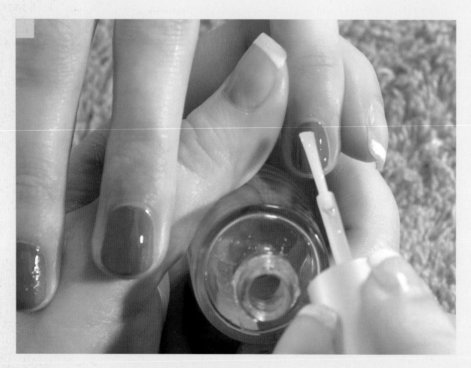

③ Top coat will give a high gloss finish but if you want to show off try a darker finish to the ends of the nails or some cleverly placed gems. Often though, classic red is the best choice and works wonders with matching accessories and lipstick!

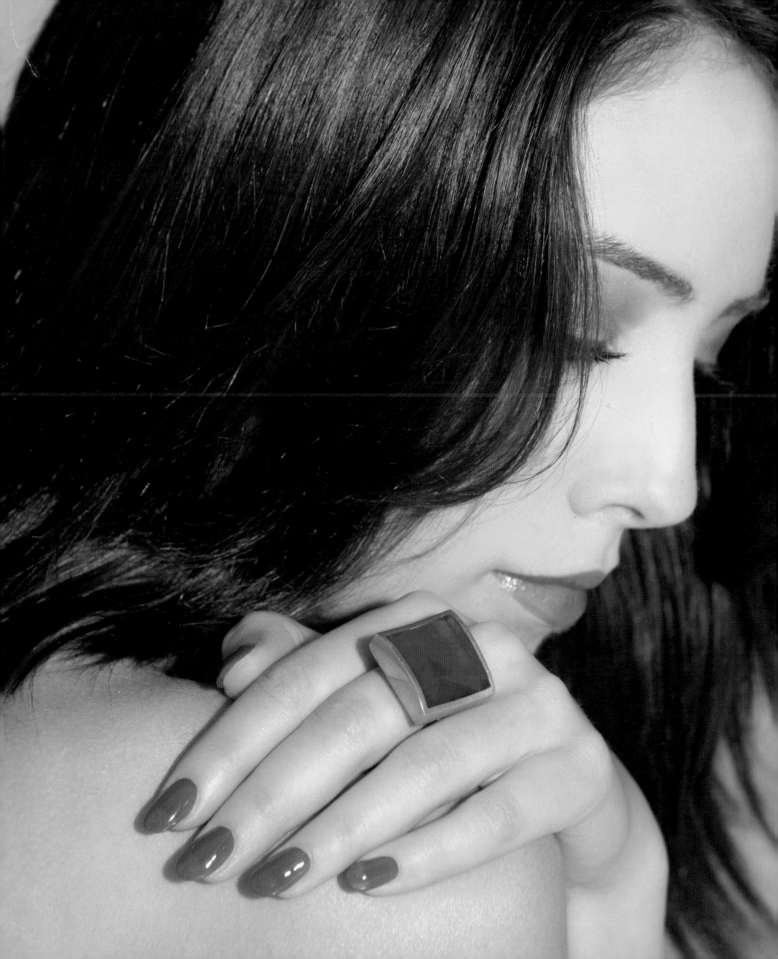

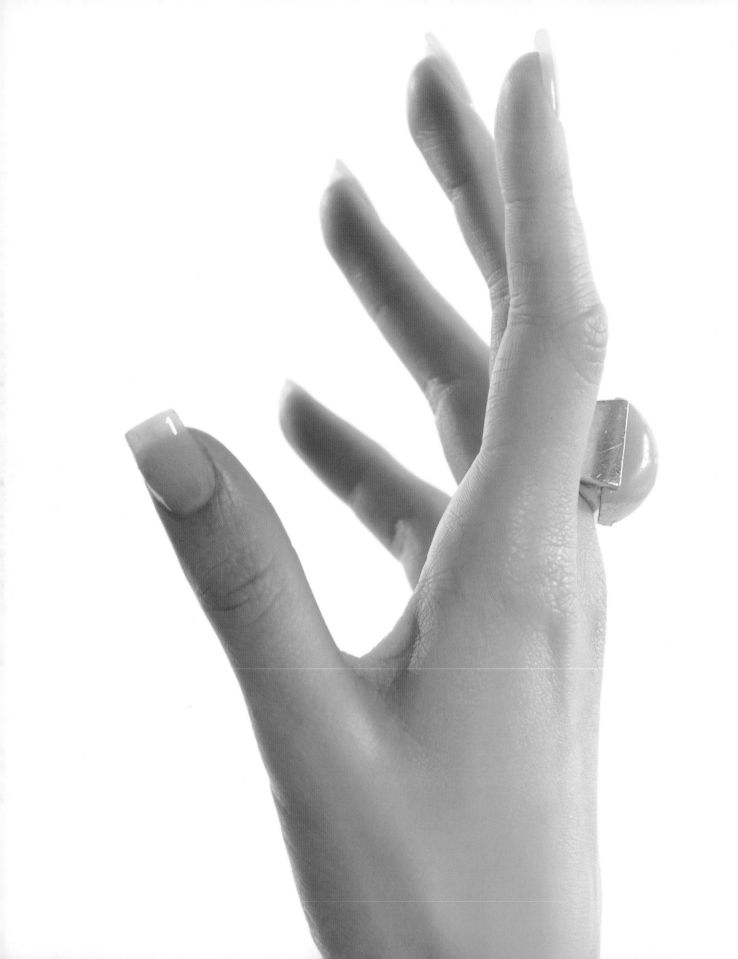

how to...

CREATE THE NEARLY NAKED LOOK

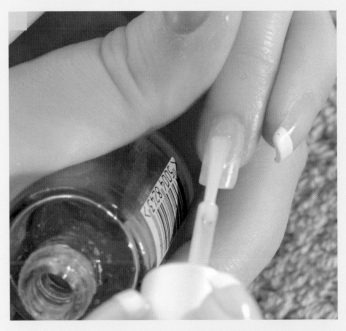

① A good basic manicure is essential as the nails must be trim and well maintained, and the cuticles nourished and not dry and flaky. After the manicure apply a clear treatment base coat and be sure to paint the tip of the nail, too.

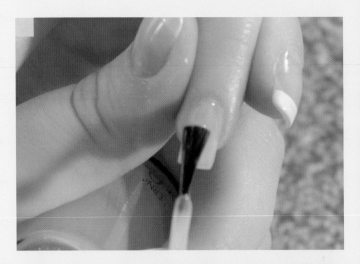

② Choose a light pink matt base varnish and apply two coats fairly liberally. If your nails are stained or yellow in tone make these coats thicker to disguise the natural tone of your nails.

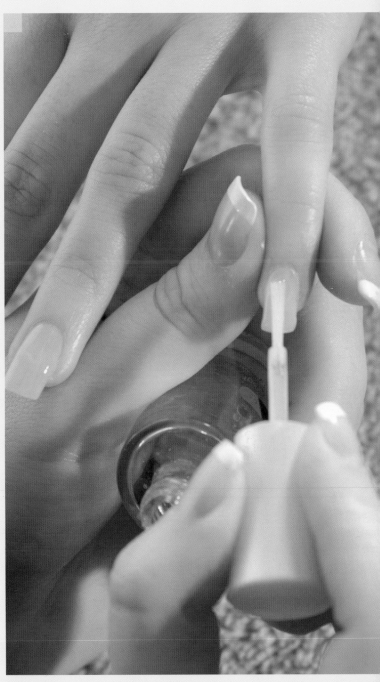

③ Finally, apply a high gloss top coat to the nails and wear them with pride! For the nearly naked look add a thin line of glitter to the tips of the nails to add a bit of sparkle to the overall result.

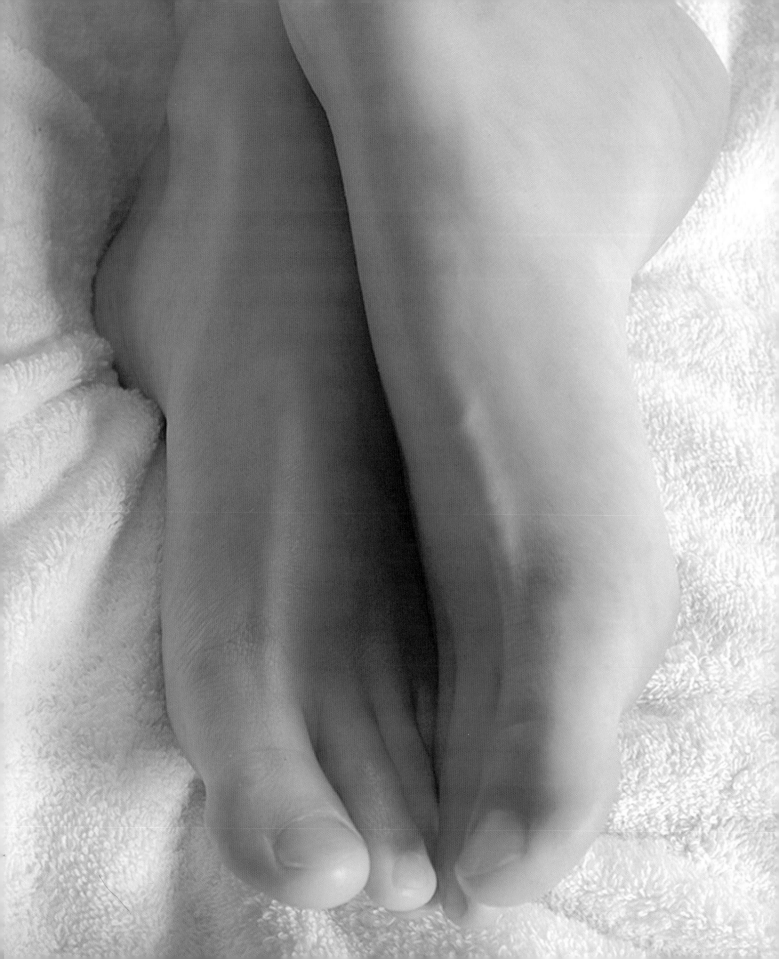

the spa

the spa

Foot and hand treatments vary enormously, from warm oils and waxes to specialised massage and the use of machinery to generate specific sensations. The market is always changing but more sophisticated treatments are now becoming really popular in nail bars in the US and Europe.

Most spa treatments involve a luxury massage with a pre-taster of a foot scrub or mask to prime the skin to accept aromatic oils. There are many variations of spa massage but all are heavenly and need to be tested out!

Thai massage

Thai foot massage is a massage of the lower legs and feet which involves hands-on stretching and massage manipulation to 're-open' sen (energy) lines, in conjunction with the use of a stick implement to stimulate the reflex points on the feet which correspond to internal organs of the body. Thai foot massage is used to promote general health and well-being. After a foot massage, therapists will often massage around the shoulders and neck to release extra tension before finishing the treatment.

This holistic treatment has been practised for many thousands of years in Asia and is very successful at de-stressing its receivers and creating a sensation of internal well-being as it concentrates on rebalancing energy within the body.

Balinese massage

This is a vigorous massage involving hot oils, essential oils for aroma and a selection of different moves to help treat stress and all of its related problems. Indonesia is made up of thousands of islands, all of which have their own different massage techniques, including Sasak, Lombok and Urat massages. They all feel wonderfully different but Balinese massage is really great for joint pain and for areas that are prone to poor circulation, such as the hands and feet. Often sea salt scrubs are also used during the massage to increase the stimulation further and really detoxify the skin.

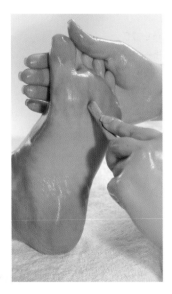
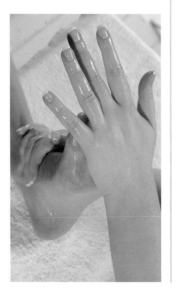
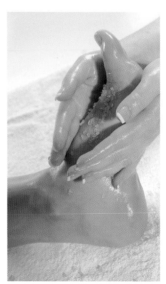
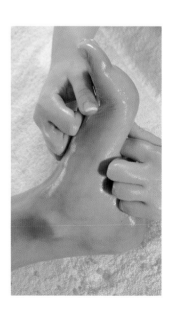

Ayurvedic massage

This massage has been used in India for thousands of years. Ayurvedic massage is very oily and it works on energy points in the body. The therapist will ask you a wide range of questions about your lifestyle, your diet and how you feel before carrying out the massage so that your treatment is completely tailored to your individual needs. Therefore every massage is different and truly unique. There are many different varieties of this specialised massage; some use powders and herbs but the traditional massage uses oils dripping on the skin and often two therapists will massage each side of the body simultaneously.

Hot stone massage

Hot volcanic basalt stones are used with fragrant essential oils to warm certain areas of the body. The therapist will then use the stones to apply a deep tissue massage to the feet and hands as well as the legs and arms. Cold or freezing stones may be used in between to stimulate the nervous and circulatory systems. As well as being relaxing the treatment is thought to be great for detoxification and aiding blood circulation in the body as well as reducing insomnia and muscle fatigue. The traditional gentle massage technique of Lomi Lomi also favours the use of hot and cold stones to add depth to a massage. Because the feet welcome firm pressure to relax them give them an extra treat with this deep tissue treatment.

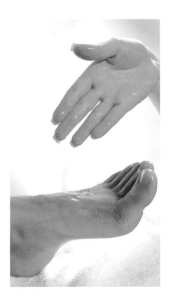
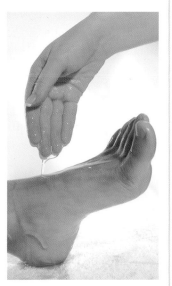
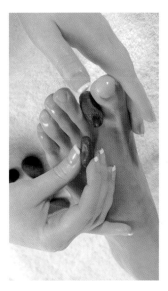
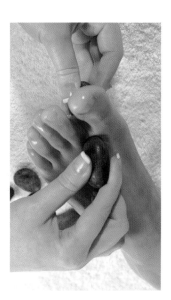

Foot bathing

Other than massage there are several other feet treats that can be performed. Foot bathing is the soaking and washing of feet in pure essences like essential oils or pure shea butter or coconut oil. The feet are rubbed in oils, spices or salt and then washed in the aromatic oils chosen by the therapist to fully cleanse the skin whilst administering a holistic treatment.

This is easy to replicate at home with your own foot spa. Simply massage your feet with an oil, preferably an aromatherapy oil, then scrub the feet with coarse sea salt before washing them in warm water and more of the same essential oils mixed with a drop of milk (this allows the essential oils to diffuse in the water properly).

Hot compress treatment

Before massage some cultures like to warm the feet to prime the skin for the absorption of essential oils. Hot towels are wrapped around the feet and are removed when they have slightly cooled. Massage oil is then applied to the feet.

This is another method that can easily be replicated at home by wetting some towels in very hot water or warming a lavender pillow in the microwave for 30 seconds. Apply to the feet and wait until they cool a little before removing and massaging the feet with essential oils. The hot cold sensations improve circulation and the warmth helps mobilise joints and ease muscle tension. This also feels great on the back of the lower legs, especially if you have been in heels all night!

Home spa

If you really haven't got the time for a professional spa treatment you can carry out your own treatments at home.

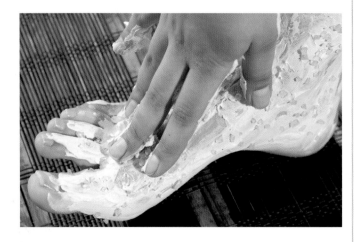

EXFOLIATE

Put a generous handful of coarse sea salt or any type of finely ground nuts in a bowl and add two drops of peppermint essential oil and two drops of lime essential oil. Make a rough paste and apply to the feet, rubbing vigorously, especially over the rough skin on the soles. Plunge your feet into a bowl of warm water and allow the salt to disperse naturally before drying the feet with a small towel.

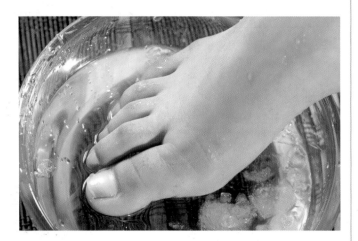

TONE

To cool or refresh hot feet in the summer plunge them into a foot spa with cold water and some ice if you're feeling really brave! Add three drops of lime oil and three drops of lemon oil to the water with a drop of milk to disperse the oils. Leave feet to soak for about 10 minutes.

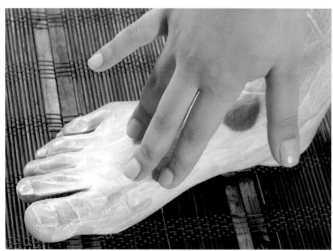

MASK

The perfect homemade mask for the feet is one which nourishes and refreshes at the same time without making a mess! In a bowl, mash an avocado with three teaspoons of olive oil, two drops of lime oil and two tablespoons of thick cream. Apply to the feet and leave to soak in for 10 minutes. These nourishing and refreshing ingredients moisturise the feet and provide a wonderful aroma for you to relax to.

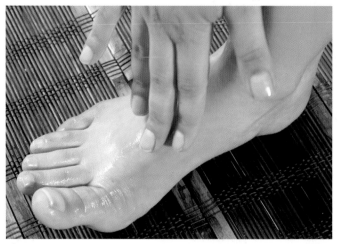

NOURISH

Moisturising with natural products is difficult so more often than not a wash-off treatment is better, however, if you really want to leave something on I would recommend simply some olive oil with a few drops of lavender and geranium essential oils. The base will nourish the feet and sink into the skin whilst the aroma essence will relax and rejuvenate your mind and soul.

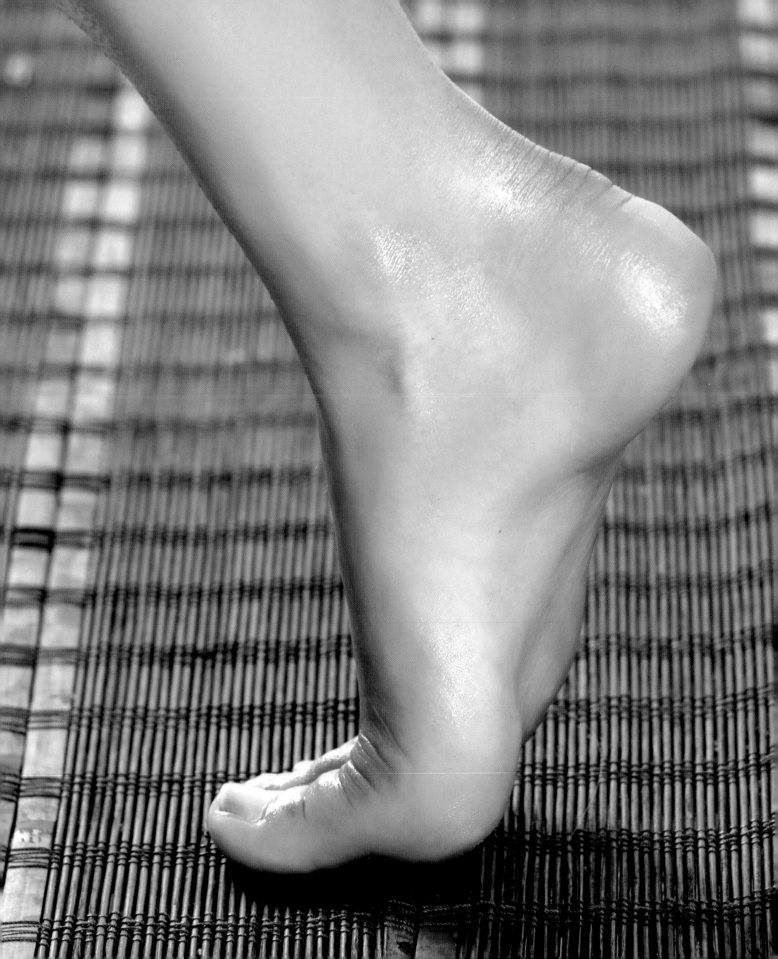

index

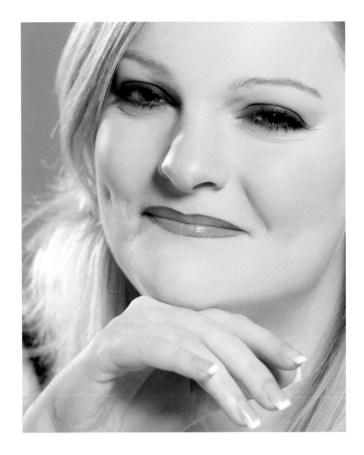

*It is always daunting writing about just one subject,
in this case nails. With fashion changes and modern
chic there is always plenty of information to pen,
however, I could not have completed one single page
without the help and guidance of my amazing editor,
Corinne, and the superb photography of Paul West.
The models who gave their time and energy to produce
such lovely pictures and finally to Elliot for his patience
and endless moral support.*

Thank you all.